The Johns Hopkins University School of Medicine Curriculum for the Twenty-first Century

Edited by

Catherine D. De Angelis, M.D.

*Professor of Pediatrics and Vice Dean
   for Academic Affairs and Faculty
The Johns Hopkins University School of Medicine
Baltimore, Maryland*

The Johns Hopkins University Press
Baltimore and London

© 1999 The Johns Hopkins University Press
All rights reserved. Published 1999
Printed in the United States of America on acid-free paper

Johns Hopkins Paperbacks edition, 2000
9 8 7 6 5 4 3 2 1

The Johns Hopkins University Press
2715 North Charles Street
Baltimore, Maryland 21218-4363
www.press.jhu.edu

Library of Congress Cataloging-in-Publication Data
will be found at the end of this book.
A catalog record for this book
is available from the British Library.

ISBN 0-8018-6350-3 (pbk.)

Contents

Foreword

The publication of this curriculum is a proud moment for the Johns Hopkins University School of Medicine. At the turn of the century, this school of medicine created the first rigorous, science-based medical curriculum in the nation. The curriculum was emulated by most medical schools and became the standard for medical education in this century. When I assumed the position of dean in 1990, the dawn of Johns Hopkins's second century was approaching. It had become clear to me that the curriculum, while basically sound, had to be revisited with a view to the demands and responsibilities of a new era. With the help of a grant from the Robert Wood Johnson Foundation and with extensive review and input from faculty, staff, and students under the direction of Catherine D. De Angelis, M.D., the school's curriculum had undergone a complete restructuring.

When I gave Dr. De Angelis and her committee its charge, I suggested that our basic philosophy of medical education must be directed not toward creating a neurosurgeon, a family practitioner, a cardiologist, or a general pediatrician but toward creating an undifferentiated "stem cell" physician who is so well prepared that he or she is fully capable of taking any career path after medical school. Every indication is that our goal is being met. The new curriculum is preparing students for the demands and responsibilities of a new era of medicine, science, and medical arts.

The reform of the Johns Hopkins curriculum truly has been a team effort, marked by schoolwide participation and a great sense of collegiality, mission, and commonality of purpose. The effort has benefited from the dedication and creative genius of hundreds of individuals, too many to name. Many of the leaders of this effort are contributors to this volume.

To all who have participated in the conception and execution of the new Johns Hopkins curriculum, and to the generations of students who will benefit from this work, this book is a small monument. It represents their commitment to sustaining the noble history of the Johns Hopkins University School of Medicine as a model of its kind.

Michael M. E. Johns, M.D.
Executive Vice President for Health Affairs
The Robert W. Woodruff Health Sciences Center
Atlanta, Georgia

Preface

The common goal of all manuals and textbooks is to impart knowledge. The general goal of this book is to describe how one school of medicine changed its curriculum from a very traditional, faculty-oriented model to a student-oriented model based on adult learning strategies.

The book is divided into ten chapters. Chapter 1 provides a brief history of undergraduate medical education at Johns Hopkins from the Flexner Report to the present. It outlines how over the more than one hundred years that the school has existed, the faculty approached education in the context of their times.

Chapter 2 provides an overview of the entire process involved in the curriculum change, which was implemented with the entering class in September 1992. It puts the next eight chapters in perspective as each relates to the whole curriculum. Many of the behind-the-scenes negotiations, discussions, frustrations, and successes are described in this chapter.

Chapter 3 describes how the teaching of first-year basic science advanced from a department-based, individual course structure to an interdepartmentally based, modular structure. Chapter 4 describes how the structure of the second year progressed from four separate courses to an interrelated course structure that is based on organ systems.

Chapter 5 describes a completely new, four-year longitudinal Physician and Society course that derived from two separate short courses in the history of medicine and bioethics, which had been taught in the first year. This course is the only one of its kind—a four-year, coordinated course that is based on the fundamentals of bioethics, and spans the fields of history, art, literature, economics, law, and sociology.

Chapter 6 describes a new curriculum for medical informatics and support services for computer-based education. The use of network information systems is vital to any advanced educational initiative, and this chapter describes one approach to the issue.

Chapter 7 describes a course in which students spend time, over the course of their first year, in the offices of community-based private practitioners. The purpose is not to teach the students clinical skills but to socialize them to the world of the practicing physician.

Chapter 8 describes curriculum reform in the clinical years, with special emphasis on the development and implementation of a new course in ambulatory general internal medicine.

Chapter 9 provides some early information on the evaluation of the general curriculum, specific courses, and the students. Finally, chapter 10 provides some general conclusions about the process and implementation of the changed curriculum, and a brief discussion of its outcome.

The overall purpose is to enable the reader to gain practical knowledge that he or she can use in changing any component of a medical curriculum, or an entire medical curriculum.

Contributors

DIANE M. BECKER, Sc.D., Associate Professor, Department of Medicine, and Director, Center for Health Promotion, Johns Hopkins University School of Medicine, Baltimore, Maryland

GERT H. BRIEGER, M.D., Ph.D., William H. Welch Professor and Director, History of Science, Medicine, and Technology, Johns Hopkins University School of Medicine, Baltimore, Maryland

LEON GORDIS, M.D., Associate Dean for Admissions and Academic Affairs, Professor, Department of Pediatrics, and Co-Director, "Physician and Society," Johns Hopkins University School of Medicine; and Professor of Epidemiology, Johns Hopkins University School of Hygiene and Public Health, Baltimore, Maryland

H. FRANKLIN HERLONG, M.D., Associate Dean of Medical Student Affairs, and Associate Professor, Department of Medicine, Johns Hopkins University School of Medicine, Baltimore, Maryland

K. JOSEPH HURT, Medical Student, Johns Hopkins University School of Medicine, Baltimore, Maryland

LANGFORD KIDD, M.D., F.R.C.P., Professor, Department of Pediatrics, Johns Hopkins University School of Medicine, Baltimore, Maryland

MICHAEL J. KLAG, M.D., Associate Professor, Department of Medicine, and Director, Division of General Internal Medicine, Johns Hopkins University School of Medicine, Baltimore, Maryland

HAROLD P. LEHMANN, M.D., Ph.D., Director, Office of Medical Informatics Education, and Assistant Professor, Department of Pediatrics, Johns Hopkins University School of Medicine, Baltimore, Maryland

NANCY RYAN LOWITT, M.D., Ed.M., Former Coordinator, "Introduction to

Clinical Medicine," Johns Hopkins University School of Medicine. Currently Associate Dean for Graduate and Continuing Medical Education, University of Maryland School of Medicine, Baltimore, Maryland

LUCY A. MEAD, Sc.M., Research Associate, Department of Medicine, Johns Hopkins University School of Medicine, Baltimore, Maryland

THOMAS D. POLLARD, M.D., Professor and President, Salk Institute for Biological Studies, La Jolla, California

HENRY M. SEIDEL, M.D., Professor Emeritus, Department of Pediatrics, and Co-Director, "Physician and Society," Johns Hopkins University School of Medicine, Baltimore, Maryland

JOHN H. SHATZER, Ph.D., Director, Office of Medical Education Services, and Assistant Professor, Division of Biomedical Information Services, Johns Hopkins University School of Medicine, Baltimore, Maryland

PATRICIA A. THOMAS, M.D., F.A.C.P., Assistant Professor, Department of Medicine, and Director, Ambulatory Clerkship in Medicine, Johns Hopkins University School of Medicine, Baltimore, Maryland

VICTOR VELCULESCU, Medical Student, Johns Hopkins University School of Medicine, Baltimore, Maryland

CHARLES M. WIENER, M.D., Assistant Professor, Department of Medicine, and Course Director, "Human Pathophysiology," Johns Hopkins University School of Medicine, Baltimore, Maryland

The Johns Hopkins University
School of Medicine Curriculum
for the Twenty-first Century

1

A Brief History of the Johns Hopkins Medical Curriculum

Gert H. Brieger, M.D.

The beginning of Johns Hopkins medical education just over a century ago was a bold, and at the same time singularly naive, departure.[1] It was bold because few had faith that such a rigorous, nontraditional program would attract any students. It was naive because science, to which the new course of studies was securely bound, was not yet well established in American medicine, indeed, was virtually unknown in American medical schools.

To begin this brief history of curricular developments in Johns Hopkins medicine, it is important to describe just what it was that we may call a Johns Hopkins model.[2] The model, of course, must be viewed in the context of American medical schools circa 1890.[3] Improvements were then beginning to occur in a few medical schools, such as Harvard and the University of Michigan and a few others, both eastern and western. Most of the country's medical schools were still of the proprietary type—that is, they were literally owned by the faculty and had budgets that were not controlled by the universities of which they were nominally a part. Most of the schools had only meager laboratory facilities, their students had only limited access to patients in hospitals or clinics, and most of the instruction was by lecture or demonstration. The medical school "year" often was not much more than four months long. If a student was fortunate in the choice of a preceptor, the apprenticeship that accompanied the didactic teaching in the medical schools was a useful means of learning some of the practical aspects of taking care of patients. But most young physicians learned to take care of patients when they embarked on their own as practitioners after two or three years of medical schooling.

Dr. John Shaw Billings, an architect of both the physical and the intellectual edifices that would come to symbolize Johns Hopkins medicine, made quite clear to the trustees of the newly founded university the importance of medicine in the

1

overall scheme of the university. The new medical school should not carry coals to Newcastle, Billings believed. Instead, he urged the university to provide a kind of medical education that was then not to be found in the United States. The new medical school, Billings wrote, should educate not just practitioners of medicine, but practitioners "fitted to make research." They should increase the stock of our medical knowledge. "I do not mean," Billings hastened to add in his 1877 lecture, "that full blown professors are to be produced, but that the graduates shall be men who can, when occasion demands, tell what they know, and why or how they know it."[4] Little did he or the other founders of the medical school realize that not all of the graduates were destined to be males.

The opening of the medical school in 1893, four years after the Johns Hopkins Hospital received its first patients, was delayed because the university lacked the funds to establish the kind of medical school that had been envisioned. Only with the action of a powerful committee of women who raised the required $500,000 could the medical school finally begin to admit its first class of students.

The bulk of the women's fund came from Mary E. Garrett, one of the active Baltimore members of the committee. Her close friend M. Carey Thomas, dean at Bryn Mawr College and its future president—and, like Garrett, a daughter of a Johns Hopkins trustee—was the moving spirit behind the conditions the Women's Fund Committee attached to its gift: the entering students had to have the equivalent of a full college education, including biology, chemistry, and physics, as well as a reading knowledge of French and German. Similar academic requirements had been discussed by the Advisory Board of the Medical Faculty and so came as much less of a surprise than the second condition of the gift: women had to be accepted on the same basis that men were.

Garrett and her friends did not expect that an equal number of women and men be admitted but insisted that the criteria for admission of men and women be the same. Carey Thomas had earlier been refused admission to the graduate division of the university (even though her father, Dr. James Carey Thomas, had been a close personal friend of Johns Hopkins and a member of the university's Board of Trustees), because the university did not admit women. But in 1893, the women who were instrumental in the opening of the medical school were not merely acting vindictively. Although the Women's Medical College existed at the time in Baltimore, few regular medical schools admitted female students. The women's committee wanted to be certain that all of the students, especially the women, were properly prepared to be successful students of medicine. Of the eighteen members of the first class, three were women.

The men who founded the Johns Hopkins University School of Medicine incorporated into its curriculum various elements of the European methods of education that they had witnessed during their own training. The teaching of the basic sciences in Baltimore was heavily influenced by the German model. The clinical sciences were taught in a way that blended British and Continental models. We can summarize the basic principles of this new medical education as follows:

1. The requirements for admission were increased. As already noted, students had first to complete a college degree that included courses in chemistry, physics, and biology. A reading knowledge of French and German were also prerequisites. Thus, medical education was to be graduate education, and as we shall see, there would be some confusion about this point in later years.

2. The lectures and demonstrations that so burdened the German medical curriculum and that of the other American schools were reduced to a minimum and supplemented by seminars, laboratory teaching, and direct contact with patients. The students were taken out of the lecture rooms and amphitheater and into the clinics and hospital wards.

3. All instruction was given by men who were actively engaged in research in their respective fields. Very few local practitioners became members of the early Johns Hopkins faculty. The professors of the preclinical subjects were full-time teachers, and they were adequately paid so that they did not have to engage in the practice of medicine. This was a new departure, and the fact that very few Baltimore physicians were appointed to the staff, of course, did not help town-gown relationships.

4. The medical course lasted for four years, and each academic year was nine months long. The first two years were devoted to the basic sciences, the latter two to the clinical specialties.

5. Spoon feeding and quizzes were generally abolished. The students were treated as adults and given great freedom in organizing their medical studies.

6. A key ingredient of the Johns Hopkins model was the very close relationship between the hospital and the medical school. Although the Johns Hopkins Hospital was not the very first university hospital, it was the largest and most active teaching institution of its kind. It thus gave the school of medicine an immense advantage from the beginning. More than half of the curriculum time has always been devoted to clinical education. Thus, the hospital has been a key factor in whatever success the medical school has achieved.

7. Finally, the model begun at Johns Hopkins included a university basis for medical education. The school of medicine did not merely have a nominal relationship to the university. Johns Hopkins, before his death in 1873, stipulated to his trustees that the university would include a medical school that would have a close relationship to the hospital he also endowed. Thus, from the beginning,

the medical school was an integral part of the university and shared its academic ethos. This was a relationship that in subsequent decades we have come to take for granted, but it was not the norm in 1893.

Among the founding faculty of the Johns Hopkins University School of Medicine there was a shared vision of what a good medical education should be. This vision attracted a group of like-minded men to the faculty to carry out that vision. Such a consensus has been far more difficult for succeeding generations to achieve, which may help to explain why recurrent curriculum committees on the local scene and repeated commissions of inquiry on a national scale have identified similar problems but have found few permanent solutions. Medical faculty members of the late twentieth century often give their primary allegiance to their disciplinary peers in national and international specialty or scientific societies rather than to their schools, universities, or even departments. Perhaps true improvements in medical education will be possible only when faculty switch some of their allegiance back to the medical colleges from the invisible colleges where it now so often resides.

The application of a university ideal to the professional education for medicine provided by Johns Hopkins and a few like-minded schools at the turn of the century validated the general principle that the main functions of a university and a university medical school were to transmit to a new generation of students the best of the learning that was available and to add to the store of knowledge by fostering research.[5]

This early period of Johns Hopkins medicine was remembered by Dr. Lewis Weed, an anatomist and himself a later dean of the school:

> The eighteen-nineties for the first time saw American schools of medicine as integral, rather than remote, parts of universities, with full-time instructors in the pre-clinical subjects and with a university point of view. This university point of view may be summarized as one in which research is looked upon as an opportunity, as a function of every instructor. In such a school, a teacher must consider his phase of medical instruction not as a finished subject to be presented by didactic methods, but as one constantly advancing. In this advance the teacher must be a participant, if only in a very small way. This attitude of investigation is essential for the establishment of medical education on a true academic basis: research and teaching are indissolubly blended.[6]

The history of the curriculum of the Johns Hopkins University School of Medicine is both unique and typical for American medical schools of the last hundred years. It is unique because at the school's inception in 1893, a remarkably talented, young, and innovative faculty (William Osler at age forty-four was the "old man" of the group) began with a blank slate. While the new venture in medical education in Baltimore, where six other medical schools were already teaching medical students, had no traditions to overcome, a second unique aspect of its history is that in the subsequent century the successors of the original faculty had always to measure themselves against the high standards and unique accomplishments of the founders.

At Johns Hopkins, as in all other medical schools, a dean or the faculty was periodically moved to assess the state of the curriculum by means of committees, reports, and faculty discussions. Typically, changes were minor in nature, and even reform measures that had wide faculty and administration approval were implemented only slowly. Conservation of the best of the old was highly valued. "If it ain't broke, don't fix it"—this philosophy was as often encountered at Johns Hopkins as at any other medical school.

An overall glance at the history of curriculum reform at Johns Hopkins reveals an interesting trend that can be divided into periods of about thirty years. The first serious review of the curriculum came in 1921, just about three decades after the school opened. Major changes in the curriculum were proposed in 1927 and again in 1957, and the present changes described in this book began with an eighteen-month review ending in 1987. Since the mid-1950s, there have been some major and many minor attempts to reform the curriculum. For the sake of brevity, I will not discuss all of them as extensively as I do the 1957 and 1987 attempts.

In the years after the opening of the Johns Hopkins University School of Medicine in 1893, what little change occurred in the curriculum was mainly by accretion. Slowly but surely, as medical knowledge expanded, so did the material presented to the students. The number of hours spent in lectures slowly increased, and free time was reduced. The school that began with the motto, "Learning by Doing" steadily went down a path that led to increasingly passive learning by its students. Dr. William H. Welch's early warning that medical education is not completed at the medical school was not always kept in mind. Nor was his concise philosophy of teaching always heeded as the years passed: "No subject should be taught as if the student were to become a specialist in it. The teaching must be simple and clear. The problems that are of most interest to the teacher are often not those with which the student need concern himself."[7]

When the school was not yet two decades old, it received accolades from the Flexner Report (1910).[8] Abraham Flexner, an 1889 graduate of the Johns Hopkins University's undergraduate program, but not himself a medical graduate, inspected all of the 162 medical schools of the United States and Canada in 1909–10. In his report, the Flexner model for medical education was derived from the Johns Hopkins model of William Welch, William Osler, and Franklin

P. Mall. While Osler and Mall disagreed on the issue of a full-time clinical faculty, the Johns Hopkins model that I described above is what impressed Flexner and Henry Pritchett, the president of the Carnegie Foundation, which was the sponsor of the survey of North American medical schools undertaken by Flexner in 1909–10.

In the Flexner Report and its introduction, Flexner and Pritchett stressed that the issues of medical education needed to be discussed not merely from the point of view of medicine but as a part of education more generally. Thus, Flexner stressed that medical students should have a proper preparatory education in the basic sciences of chemistry, physics, and biology; that medical teachers should combine instruction with research; that medical faculties should devote their entire time to teaching and research, for which they should receive sufficient salary so as not to be dependent on the income from medical practice; and that medical schools should be a part of a parent university and not a property of the faculty. If all of this sounds familiar, it is because it became the norm for academic medicine in the decades following 1910. At the time of the Flexner Report, only a handful of schools embraced most or all of the features stressed by Flexner.

For Flexner, the Johns Hopkins University School of Medicine was the ideal model of what a medical school should be. He wrote in his report that at Johns Hopkins the laboratory facilities "are in every respect unexcelled. As the institution has been from the beginning on a graduate basis, teaching and research have been always equally prominent in its activities."[9] About the clinical facilities Flexner proclaimed that "the Johns Hopkins Hospital and Dispensary provide practically ideal opportunities."[10]

Thus, Flexner held up Johns Hopkins as the ideal to which all medical schools should aspire. And so, in just two decades, Johns Hopkins medicine was able to achieve what one of its principle designers, Dr. John Shaw Billings, had hoped for it: it had become a model of its kind.

In 1921 a committee of five senior professors met seventeen times to consider the status of the school. Mindful of the ever-increasing quantity of medical knowledge (a problem articulated in all periods of the history of medicine since the eighteenth century), the committee was concerned that without proper care the curriculum could become "lopsided." In some subjects, they admitted in their final report, this was already apparent, and they noted that too much required instruction had crept into the curriculum.[11]

The committee suggested that there should be a minimum of required courses in the major subjects and that an extensive elective system should be developed. Students were to be stimulated to do research, and the heads of the departments should once again assume personal charge of their introductory courses. All of these recommendations merely show how far the curriculum had strayed since the school's early days. An additional recommendation was that the number of students admitted to the first year be reduced from ninety to seventy-five. Tuition was to be raised from $250 to $300 per year to offset the money lost by reducing the number of students. A class of seventy-five was admitted beginning in 1924.

In the years after 1921, a series of committees continued to wrestle with the problems of an increasingly crowded and rigid curriculum. When the medical school opened in 1893, four years had seemed to be ample time to cover all the medical subjects. Thirty to forty years later, the specter of an overcrowded curriculum had become reality.

It was not only at Johns Hopkins that the curriculum had become, by the 1920s, overcrowded and burdened by lectures. Looking at American medical schools in 1925, a mere fifteen years after his famous study of 1910, Abraham Flexner was shocked and disappointed to learn that medical students across the country followed a lock-step routine and that, unfortunately, Johns Hopkins was no exception. "The students were grouped," Flexner wrote, "in fixed classes . . . followed in fixed order, day by day the same subject for the same length of time. . . . From 8:30 to 1:00, from 2:00 to 4:30, all students in their respective classes pursued an identical routine. . . . Anything more alien to the spirit of scientific or modern medicine or to university life could hardly be contrived."[12]

All over the world, Flexner complained, medical curricula were burdened by the inclusion of too many subjects and too much material. "It is indeed no paradox to assert," Flexner added, "that though medicine can be learned, it cannot be taught. The student must throw himself eagerly and intelligently into the quest. He must want to learn."[13] By the time the curriculum at Johns Hopkins was reviewed in the 1920s, the faculty agreed with what Flexner had written in his 1925 book.

In 1923, when Dr. Lewis Weed became dean, he formed a committee on both the curriculum and educational policy. Weed had been a member of the small group that looked at the curriculum in 1921. As he recalled a decade later, what had been happening in all medical schools after the turn of the century, in response to the widening scope and depth of scientific advances, was a steady increase in the number of required subjects and required hours in the four-year curriculum.

At Johns Hopkins in 1926, the Committee on Educational Policy began its report to the dean and the advisory board by restating what had been very clear to the founding faculty in 1893: "If the study of medicine is to be considered of a true professional nature, the School of Medicine should place its courses of instruction upon as thorough a graduate basis as is compatible with the training of students for a profession."[14] The report recommended that the number of hours of required instruction be decreased, thus allowing for more free time. The committee further urged that the school allow students to study for periods of time at other institutions, and that students be allowed to discontinue their regular medical studies to devote a year or more to special studies in any subject.[15]

These suggestions echoed Weed's philosophy of medical education, which he expressed in a commencement address at Cornell in 1929 and at the opening exercises of the new Duke University School of Medicine in 1930. He noted that one of the important tenets of medical education was "the idea that for the greatest individual development, the student must be granted utmost freedom in choice of work, the required courses being limited to the minimum and the optional work being as free as possible."[16]

At Cornell, Weed told the medical graduates that it was the task of the medical teacher to avoid turning out students who were merely skillful practitioners. "Such medical graduates would leave their schools lacking the most desirable attitude of mind towards medical problems and without an equally desirable interest in the humanistic side of medicine."[17] Medical schools, Weed staunchly believed, should "create and foster the inquiring student of medicine."[18] And it was in this spirit that the reforms discussed at Johns Hopkins between 1921 and 1926 were formalized by the Advisory Board of the Medical Faculty in 1927. The trimester system was changed to the quarter system, about half the students' time was available for freely chosen elective courses, and examinations were given at the end of the second and fourth years.[19]

Although the recommendations of the committees of the early 1920s were undertaken with the usual fanfare of a "new" curriculum, it was not long before critical voices began to be heard. Among the most articulate of these was that of a young professor of pathology, Dr. Arnold R. Rich. In a forty-page report published in 1931, Rich pulled no punches.[20] He emphasized that expert teachers and good students were far more important to the enterprise of medical education than were any clever arrangements of the curriculum. The curriculum should be planned for the average student, Rich said, because the very gifted will flourish in any case.

Rich believed in treating students as adults, but in light of the inadequacies of their preliminary education he did not have confidence in their ability to know what was best for them and how best to achieve those ends. Thus, he questioned the liberal elective policy that the school had adopted. He argued against the notion that medical education was truly a graduate education. A graduate student in the true meaning of that term, Rich maintained, "is one who pursues advanced work in a particular field after having acquired a satisfactory preliminary familiarity with the basic principles of that field."[21] Unlike graduate students in the humanities or the social sciences, "the student entering medical school approaches a field with which he has not the slightest preliminary acquaintance except for the slender connection between college zoology and human anatomy and that between college chemistry and physiological chemistry."[22]

The goals of the medical curriculum, Rich believed, were relatively simple ones. The curriculum should provide a foundation of the basic principles of medicine upon which clinical experience could rest. Each student should have the opportunity to develop according to individual talents and desires. And the curriculum should be as brief as possible, so that the student could proceed from passive to active learning as quickly as possible. Rich, along with many in medical education since the early years of the century, believed that the formal period of education from high school to medical practice was far too long and wasted precious years during which a young physician could be the most creative. This was an argument that would play a major role in the next major curriculum revision in the mid-1950s.

With the glowing exception of the original pioneering reform of medical education in 1893, curricular changes at Johns Hopkins must be viewed in the context of changes going on in the other medical schools. This is especially true for the early 1950s, when there was much discussion of the fundamental alterations in the way in which medical courses were arranged and taught at Case Western Reserve University in Cleveland. Similarly, in the 1980s, the widespread discussions of the GPEP Report[23] and Harvard's New Pathway Program, the latter taking what recently had been pioneered at the University of New Mexico and at McMaster University in Canada, also influenced many schools, including Johns Hopkins, once again to look inward at their own form and methods of medical education.

In 1952, with the return to Johns Hopkins of Dr. W. Barry Wood as professor of microbiology and vice president of medical affairs, and the appointment of a new committee to consider medical education at Johns Hopkins, chaired by Dr. John C. Whitehorn, professor of psychiatry, a process of major reform that would take the better part of the 1950s to implement began in earnest. With the perceived growth of medical knowledge in those days when cortisone and the antibiotics were coming into wide use, Whitehorn noted that "it has required restraint, judgement, and courage to curb the tendency toward instructional elephantiasis."[24] Whitehorn was ahead of his time in pointing out the changing economic practices that had increased the number of patients covered by insurance and therefore decreased the number of indigent patients who were available for the traditional ward teaching.

Wood, picking up a theme from Rich's 1931 report, noted that "the most serious defect in present-day medical education is the excessive number of years required to train a physician. As knowledge in medical science has increased, the combined undergraduate and post graduate medical course has become longer and longer."[25]

But it was not merely the length of medical education that was at issue for American medical schools during these heady postwar years. As research money became more plentiful for the biomedical sciences, it did so also for the general sciences and engineering. Leaders of academic medicine at Johns Hopkins and elsewhere began to note that the best students were increasingly being attracted to other fields, a trend only exacerbated by the launch of *Sputnik* in 1957. Streamlining medical education, many believed, might help to attract more of the better students back to medicine.

In a ten-page memorandum to the entire medical faculty in 1957, Wood described the new program devised by the Whitehorn committee, and he fully discussed the problems of medical education that gave rise to the proposals. The length of medical studies not only discouraged some good applicants but also forced some medical graduates into private practice before they gained adequate post-M.D. training, or discouraged them from embarking upon research careers.[26]

The Whitehorn committee also paid specific attention to the difficulties that students encountered in the transition from college to medical school, the transition from the preclinical to the clinical curriculum in the medical school, and the transition from medical school to house staff, all of which were key issues in the reform discussions of the 1960s and 1970s. Regarding the first transition, Wood noted the deficiencies caused by the sharp separation between the collegiate experience and the medical school. Using a good Cold War metaphor, he claimed that "the curriculum for medical students has always been virtually cut in two by an 'iron curtain' which drops precipitously at the end of college. Once he enters medical school, the prospective physician is expected to leave behind his interests in the humanities and social sciences in order to devote himself exclusively to the study of medicine. Divorced so abruptly and so completely from the pursuit of a general education, he all too frequently loses interest in everything except the technical requirements of his chosen profession. With such a system in vogue, it is not surprising that many American physicians, though technically competent, appear deficient in their historical and humanistic understanding, even in matters closely related to health."[27]

To reduce the barriers between the collegiate and medical phases of education, to improve teaching and heighten interest in the premedical and preclinical sciences, and to incorporate the social sciences and humanities for a better understanding of modern health problems, the Johns Hopkins proposal for a markedly revised program actually went into effect for a portion of the class in 1959.[28]

The revised program allowed twenty-five students to pursue a general education in college for two years and then to enter a five-year medical school program. The first year was divided between the arts and sciences campus, where the students took courses in social science or humanities and a physics course, and the medical school, where members of the preclinical faculty taught advanced chemistry and genetics.

The program allowed students to proceed from high school to residency in seven rather than the customary eight years, encouraged the students to retain an interest in the liberal arts while they studied medicine, and improved instruction in the main premedical sciences by gearing them more toward the problems of medicine. A change implemented for the entire medical school class was a required year-long course in the history of medicine in year 2, the first year of the traditional preclinical curriculum, which was the year in which the twenty-five early admission students joined the bulk of the class admitted after college graduation.

The five-year program ran for twenty years, until 1979, when a new program in human biology began. Both the new program and the old were funded mainly by a grant from the Commonwealth Fund. Of interest from the historian's perspective is the paucity of documentation for the ending of the twenty-year program known as Year V. While there were many internal documents and several published reports from the 1950s, the end in 1979 left virtually no trace.

The Commonwealth Fund had supported American medical education since the 1920s.[29] In the 1970s its president, Dr. Carleton B. Chapman, a former medical school dean at Dartmouth, was particularly interested in the collaboration between all parts of universities to provide a better integration between the premedical and preclinical phases of the student's education. The directors of the fund hoped to stimulate the faculties in the arts and sciences and those in medicine to plan effectively for a curriculum that required premedical and medical education to be considered as a continuum, not as a series of unconnected steps in the students' path to a medical career. By the 1970s, Chapman wrote, the content and the boundaries of the biological sciences were vastly different than they were in Flexner's day. The premedical science requirements had not been revised for more than half a century, though during that span there were great changes in the natural, biologic, and behavioral sciences.[30]

The Human Biology Program, like its predecessor the Year V Program, was designed to shorten by one year the usual eight-year education (four in college and four in medical school) of medical students. The intent of the Human Biology Program was to provide an even closer link between courses in the medical school and those in biology in the school of arts and sciences.

The Human Biology Program was dropped after three years as funding ran out and the number and quality of applicants decreased. The program actually became a roadblock to curricular changes in the school of medicine because of difficulties in meshing undergraduate and medical school courses.

It is quite natural to focus on innovation and new methods of education. Americans, being a "new" society, have always equated that which is new with that which is good. Perhaps—like death, which in medicine we do not like to talk about and often consider as a defeat—the demise of a curricular innovation is also surrounded by silence more than by discussion and analysis. At least in medicine we have the tradition of the clinicopathological conference. Medical education would doubtless benefit if we forced ourselves to conduct a similarly critical exercise for our educational endeavors.

A series of curriculum committees in the late 1960s and the early 1970s continued to address the usual problems of medical education, which included number of courses, free time, sequence of courses, and the coordination between them. Class size increased from 82 to 109 in 1969, and by 1980 the present class size of 120 was established.

From 1969 to 1972, curriculum committees chaired by Julius R. Krevans, associate dean for academic affairs, evaluated current programs, grappled with problems of redundance, urged greater cooperation between departments to provide interdisciplinary courses, and urged the faculty to provide a better system of student advising. A 1975/76 committee chaired by a professor of physiology, Dr. Vernon B. Mountcastle, recognized that developments in the sciences necessitated shifting from block courses in separate disciplines toward more cross-disciplinary teaching.[31] The committee's report urged new courses such as Cells and Tissues, which the basic science faculty successfully merged with an even more interdisciplinary first-year basic science curriculum described by Dr. Thomas Pollard in chapter 3 of this book.

The report submitted by the Mountcastle committee in early 1976 recognized the changes in the sciences of medicine discussed by Chapman and others at the time, and that committee also laid the groundwork for the Human Biology Program that is described above. In important ways, that committee also laid the groundwork for the changes that have continued to the present and that are the subject of this book.

The Mountcastle committee, in a letter that accompanied their report when it was transmitted to the president of the university, wrote: "We recommend a radical change in the medical curriculum, clustering molecular, cellular, and systems biology, respectively, in the first year, emphasizing pathobiology in the second year, and providing additional basic science teaching later in the curriculum. The various clusters would be planned and taught by interdepartmental faculty groups, but designated departments would have primary responsibility for individual courses."[32]

In virtually every medical school today, there exists a continuing tension between tradition and innovation. At Johns Hopkins, because of the uniqueness that characterized the medical school when it began to teach students a century ago, this tension has loomed large throughout its history. At the time of the most recent curriculum review nearly a decade ago, the committee and most of those we consulted were particularly aware of our tradition because the school of medicine and the hospital were about to embark on a centennial celebration. Yet few people realized that despite previous efforts at reform, medical education at Johns Hopkins (and elsewhere) had strayed far from the clear and relatively simple ideals of the founders.

When the curriculum review of the late 1980s began, the conventional wisdom was that despite the generally very high quality of medical care in this country, doctors were being educated and trained in response to earlier needs and as a consequence of a major list of successes stemming from a well-financed biomedical research effort. In 1984, Dr. Steven Muller, who was then the president of the Johns Hopkins University and chaired the Panel on the General Professional Education of the Physician (GPEP), wrote in the introduction to the GPEP Report, "Changes are needed now to anticipate the circumstances that are beginning to alter the practice of medicine and that today's medical students will confront in the future. The panel judges that the present system of general professional education for medicine will become increasingly inadequate unless it is revised."[33]

In Boston, the Harvard Medical School was embarking on its New Pathway Program; at first it involved only twenty-five students, but by 1987 all entering students were divided into small groups for seminar-type teaching.[34] Harvard and other North American medical schools were responding to new developments in science that were bound to change the practice of medicine. Harvard's reforms were anticipated by McMaster University in Canada and by the University of New Mexico, as already noted. The aim of all these new programs was to devise a comprehensive strategy for the entire curriculum in order to provide a program of general medical education in an age of ever-increasing subspecialization of medical practice. Since research has always been subspecialized, we can raise the question of what we have learned in the research-intensive medical schools in the last five decades about translating the specialized work of the medical teachers for the benefit of our students.

At Johns Hopkins, an ongoing process of revisions needed to decompress the basic science years was under way by the mid-1980s. The dean, Dr. Richard S. Ross, was convinced that more than mere revision was necessary, and in 1986 he appointed a committee chaired by me and composed of seven department chairs and four members of the dean's office to undertake a full reexamination of the entire curriculum.

"Re-examination of our curriculum," Dr. Ross wrote in the charge to the committee, "is also warranted by the rapid expansion of scientific knowledge and technology, major changes in the patterns of medical care delivery, greater emphasis on ethical, social and economic issues, and the promise of preventive medicine."[35] He also urged that the school should consider major changes in the curriculum then in place. Dr. Ross further believed that change heightens an interest in teaching.

Early in its deliberations, the committee identified five basic questions: (1) Are the clinical clerkships adapting to changing patterns of medical care? (2) How do we address the problems of basic science in the clinical setting? (3) Should we allow medical education at Johns Hopkins to be merely a tunnel to the residency years? Will the requirement of something like a research project or a thesis address this problem? (4) Does the diversity of our students require some educational compromises? Should we be clearer about what kinds of students we wish to attract? Is there a place for an elite approach to medical education, when elitism is taken in the best sense of that term? (5) Is our educational experience organized as an experience for adults? How closely is this question related to the problem of class size?

Clearly, the larger question still was, Were our students becoming good physicians because of our teaching and curriculum or in spite of them? Dr. Muller, meeting with the committee, wondered at the irony of a profession that is educating people to make decisions and to intervene in an active manner, yet trains its recruits in such a passive way.

Evidence from students also revealed fairly wide dissatisfaction with the style of the education they were undergoing, not with its content. Two students wrote to the committee after a meeting with me that they understood the history of the school, and that William Osler and William Welch firmly believed that active learning was the best possible means of developing the minds of future physicians.

> Medical education at Hopkins has changed since then. Students are no longer given the opportunity to participate actively in the learning process during the preclinical years. Most of our days are spent sitting in lecture halls, and little time has been allocated for the active exchange of ideas. As a result, we who arrived at Johns Hopkins as motivated, independent, and intellectually gifted individuals, unaccustomed to learning by rote only, have become frustrated as we have found ourselves playing a passive role in our own medical educations. No longer are we expected to critically evaluate information or to ask questions, nor are we encouraged to do so. Memorization of textbooks and lecture handouts now takes precedence over understanding concepts. Learning has ceased to be fun.

Though we have adapted to the demands of medical school, successful adaptation has come at a high price. Over the past year and a half, our class has changed significantly. Questions following lectures, which used to be frequent, are now sparse. People no longer have the energy or the inclination to pursue academic topics in depth. We are now intimidated when called upon in class to speak and to reason through approaches to hypothetical clinical situations. One pathophysiology professor was surprised to find that students were remarkably adept at citing lists of features pertinent to a particular disease, but were entirely unable to recognize this same data when presented in the forms of photographs or case descriptions.[36]

Needless to say, these second-year medical students were saddened to see how they and their classmates had been changed. Their response to the educational process of the first two years of medical school is, of course, not unique to their time or to their school. I have heard very similar things in other schools for a period of several decades. This example also affirms that the problems of medical education have long been identified, but corrective measures have always proved difficult. This was also well demonstrated in a recent review of nineteen reports of medical education surveys since the Flexner Report of 1910. The author, Dr. Nicholas Christakis, found constant concerns, repeated in a litany of similar problems, seemingly unsolved over the course of this entire century.[37]

The final report of the Curriculum Review Committee of 1986/87, entitled "A Curriculum for the Second Century of Johns Hopkins Medicine," also known as the Brieger Report, contained only seven very general recommendations. Since the remainder of this book will discuss how some of these have been modified and implemented, it will be useful to include them here. Each of the seven recommendations had supporting discussion, but that will be omitted here.

1. Reorient both preclinical and clinical instruction so that students will progress beyond the mere acquisition of facts and concepts (the vocabulary and grammar of biomedical science) to a level of scientific fluency with which they can begin to think creatively about biomedical problems. Our curriculum should stimulate scientific curiosity and prepare our graduates to complete the training required to carry out original research in either a clinical or laboratory setting.

2. Organize the curriculum with the objective of presenting the material most logically and efficiently, and of emphasizing independent study and active learning. This will require major changes in our current schedule of required classes and electives, and enhanced coordination among courses.

3. Introduce a four-year, weekly, student-faculty seminar to read and evaluate original research papers. Each seminar will consist of 8–12 students, 1 basic scientist, and 1 clinician. In the first year the student will learn

how to evaluate the scientific literature critically. Advanced students will keep abreast of developments in the basic biomedical, social, and behavioral sciences and of the relevance of those developments to solving clinical problems.

4. Create a four-year, longitudinal course that in the first two years emphasizes clinical skills, epidemiology, ethics, the history of medicine, and the principles of clinical decision-making, of preventive medicine, and of the psychosocial aspects of patient care. This course will provide the basis for an appreciation of the social and biological challenges explicit in patient care, and it will introduce students to patients from the beginning of their first year. In the final two years the course will provide continuing ambulatory care teaching in appropriate settings.

5. Require original research reported in a thesis, and provide time in the curriculum for research and writing. The subject of the research may be in any area of basic science or clinical medicine, and may include topics in the social sciences, epidemiology, or the humanities as they pertain to medicine.

6. Restructure clinical clerkships to eliminate redundancies and to focus on the intellectual content of the clinical sciences. The goals of the clerkships should be re-examined with emphasis placed on: the understanding of the expected normal as well as the unexpected abnormal; clinical problem-solving; and discussion of the advances in each specific field. Since students will have substantial experience with ambulatory patient care in the four-year longitudinal course, time allotted to clerkships may be reduced.

7. Appoint a coordinator of medical education fully empowered by the Dean and the Advisory Board to implement these recommendations, to oversee the formation of a new curriculum, and to foster improved coordination among courses.

In concluding this brief survey of Johns Hopkins curricular history, it is worth noting that what medical educators have called the Johns Hopkins model is no longer unique. This may indeed be the single greatest achievement of the new medical education of 1893. We now take for granted that faculty should be recruited from the best available anywhere in the world; that students should be prepared for the study of medicine by a well-rounded liberal arts education (which includes science); and that the basis of medical practice is firmly anchored in the medical sciences. All of this seems self-evident to those engaged in the continuing efforts to improve medical education in the last years of the twentieth century. And it is ample affirmation that what was started in Baltimore and a few other places in the 1890s has had enduring qualities. Over the last hundred years, literally hundreds of curriculum committees in all American medical schools have amply demonstrated that it is especially when we have strayed from these ideals that we have had to pull ourselves back to a path that has led to many successes. It is as true in the 1990s as it was in the 1890s, in the words of William H. Welch, that the results of the system are better than the system warrants.

The last paragraph of John Stuart Mill's famous essay "On Liberty" begins with the assertion that "the worth of a state, in the long run, is the worth of the individuals composing it."[38] And we might say the same for the worth of the medical profession. It is the responsibility of the medical schools to prepare our students for the tasks of medical citizenship. It is this notion of a civic medicine, or medicine as a public service, that needs to be as implicit in a good medical education as are the virtues of science.

Although an old saw has it that changing the curriculum in a medical school is more difficult than moving a cemetery, the truth is that changes occurred in the first century of Johns Hopkins medicine and doubtless will continue in the second. Some of these changes have been major, others slow and incremental. Such has been the case in virtually all American medical schools in this century. This should not be surprising, because those who plan and execute the curriculum are the scientists and clinicians who in their own work continuously adapt their research strategies and patient care methods to the changes in science and technology.

Medicine has, since the late nineteenth century, had a secure partnership with the basic sciences of chemistry, physics, and biology. In the last four decades much ink, many dollars, and great effort have been expended to forge a similar link to the social and behavioral sciences. It was, in part at least, to strengthen this link and to take advantage of a growing knowledge of how we learn and how we ought to teach that the reforms of the mid-1950s and the late 1980s were made. It is important also to stress that curriculum reform has always implied much more than merely shifting hours or courses. Changing the context of the curriculum must be accompanied by an understanding of the philosophy behind it. That philosophy, of course, needs to take into consideration what a doctor needs to know to practice medicine today and what principles are necessary to prepare to practice the medicine of tomorrow.

William H. Welch said it succinctly in 1893 in the first catalog of the Johns Hopkins University School of Medicine: "Medical education is not completed at the medical school; it is only begun. Hence it is not only or chiefly the quantity of knowledge which the student takes with him from the school which will help him in his future work; it is also the quality of mind, the methods of work, the disciplined habit of correct reasoning, the way of looking at medical problems."[39]

The style and content of medical education today and the attitudes it fosters will determine the quality of our health care tomorrow. And an essential element of this education is enjoyment of the learning process. At Johns Hopkins we need to make learning and teaching once again the fun that they were in the early days of the medical school.

Notes

1. This was the view expressed by Abraham Flexner in his 1925 book comparing American and European medical education. A. Flexner, *Medical education: A comparative study* (New York: Macmillan, 1925), 43.

2. There is an extensive literature on the history of Johns Hopkins medicine. The standard sources are A. M. Chesney, *The Johns Hopkins Hospital and the Johns Hopkins University School of Medicine, 1867–1914,* 3 vols. (Baltimore: Johns Hopkins Press, 1943–63); T. B. Turner, *Heritage of excellence: The Johns Hopkins Medical Institutions, 1914–1946* (Baltimore: Johns Hopkins University Press, 1974); and A. M. Harvey, G. H. Brieger, S. L. Abrams, and V. A. McKusick, *A model of its kind: A centennial history of medicine at Johns Hopkins,* 2 vols. (Baltimore: Johns Hopkins University Press, 1989). All general statements about the Johns Hopkins curriculum in this chapter may be found in these sources unless otherwise indicated.

3. The best summary of the history of medical education in the United States is K. H. Ludmerer, *Learning to heal* (New York: Basic Books, 1985).

4. J. S. Billings, "Suggestions on medical education," *Bulletin of the History of Medicine* 6 (1983): 326. This article is a compilation of lectures given by Billings in 1877, shortly after the opening of the university.

5. See the references in n. 2, above; and W. H. Welch, "Some advantages of the union of medical school and university," *New England and Yale Review* 13 (1888): 145–63.

6. L. H. Weed, "Experimentation in medical education," *Southern Medical Journal* 24 (1931): 1116–21.

7. W. H. Welch, "Higher medical education and the need of its endowment," *Medical News* 65 (1894): 63–70.

8. A. Flexner, *Medical education in the United States and Canada* (New York: Carnegie Foundation for the Advancement of Teaching, 1910).

9. Ibid., 235.

10. Ibid.

11. "Report of the committee appointed to consider the status of the medical school," 1921, A. M. Chesney Medical Archives, Johns Hopkins University, Baltimore, Md. (hereafter cited as "Chesney Medical Archives").

12. A. Flexner, *Medical education: A comparative study* (New York: Macmillan, 1925), 137–38.

13. Ibid., 148.

14. "Committee on Educational Policies to Advisory Board of the Medical Faculty," 1926, p. 1, Chesney Medical Archives.

15. Ibid.

16. L. H. Weed, "Experimentation in medical education," *Southern Medical Journal* 24 (1931): 1119.

17. L. H. Weed, "Some tenets of medical education," *Bulletin of the Johns Hopkins Hospital* 45 (1929): 214.

18. Ibid.

19. Advisory Board of the Medical Faculty, minutes of special meeting, February 4, 1927, Chesney Medical Archives.

20. A. R. Rich, "Reflections on the relation of the curriculum to certain problems in medical education," *Bulletin of the Johns Hopkins Hospital* 49 (1931): 121–61.

21. Ibid., 132.

22. Ibid.

23. Association of American Medical Colleges, *Physicians for the twenty-first century: The GPEP report,* report of the Panel on the General Professional Education of the Physician and College Preparation for Medicine (Washington, D.C.: Association of American Medical Colleges, 1984).

24. J. C. Whitehorn, "Proposed study of educational objectives and program in the Johns Hopkins Medical Institutions," 1954, Chesney Medical Archives.

25. W. B. Wood Jr., "A revised program of medical education in the Johns Hopkins University," 1957, p. 1, Chesney Medical Archives.

26. Ibid.

27. Ibid.

28. T. B. Turner, "Report: The revised program of medical education in the Johns Hopkins University," *Journal of Medical Education* 34 (1959): 267–71.

29. A. M. Harvey and S. L. Abrams, *For the welfare of mankind: The Commonwealth Fund and American medicine* (Baltimore: Johns Hopkins University Press, 1986).

30. C. B. Chapman, "President's comment," in *Annual report* (New York: Commonwealth Fund, 1976); and Chapman, "President's comment," in *Annual Report* (New York: Commonwealth Fund, 1977).

31. V. B. Mountcastle et al., "Preliminary report of the Basic Science Committee concerning the arrangement of the basic science departments of the school of medicine," 1976, Chesney Medical Archives.

32. V. B. Mountcastle to President Steven Muller, 5 March 1976, Chesney Medical Archives.

33. S. Muller, "Introduction: Physicians for the twenty-first century," *Journal of Medical Education* 59 (1984): 2.

34. D. C. Tosteson, J. S. Adelstein, and S. T. Carver, eds., *New pathways to medical education: Learning to learn at Harvard medical School* (Cambridge: Harvard University Press, 1994).

35. R. S. Ross to G. H. Brieger, July 17, 1986, in author's personal files.

36. D. Ratner and D. Barton to Curriculum Review Committee of 1986/87, February 26, 1987, in author's personal files.

37. N. Christakis, "The similarity and frequency of proposals to reform U.S. medical education," *JAMA* 274 (1995): 706–11.

38. J. S. Mill, "On liberty" (1849). This essay appears in many available editions of Mill's work.

39. W. H. Welch, *Announcement of the Johns Hopkins Medical School* (Baltimore, 1893); reprinted in G. H. Brieger, *Medical America in the nineteenth century* (Baltimore: Johns Hopkins University Press, 1972), 313–30.

2

Overview

Catherine D. De Angelis, M.D.

Development of the Proposal

In July 1990, Dr. Michael Johns became the dean of the Johns Hopkins University School of Medicine. I had served on the search committee that chose him to be the dean. One of the issues with which I had plagued the candidates for the deanship was education, and especially the education of medical students. Therefore, when Dean Johns asked me to become the associate dean for academic affairs and to lead the initiative for a new curriculum, it would have been difficult to refuse his offer. He pledged his enthusiastic support for the initiative, and the president of the university, Dr. William C. Richardson, also made a special effort to convince me that a new curriculum for the school of medicine was of prime importance to him and the entire university. Therefore I accepted the position and embarked on an adventure that was to last for five years in the development and implementation, and a lifetime in my memories.

The goal of this chapter is to provide as much information as possible so that the reader can understand the intricacies of designing and implementing a new curriculum, at least at one institution. While no two institutions or curricula are exactly the same, many of the major issues and problems are essentially the same. I will cover the areas about which I have received the most inquiries over the past six years.

The Brieger Report

I had been vaguely aware of the Brieger Report (the final report of the Curriculum Review Committee of 1986/87, entitled "A Curriculum for the Second Century of Johns Hopkins Medicine"), discussed in chapter 1, and of a preliminary planning project for curricular change (entitled "Preparing Physicians for the Future: A Program in Medical Education") that had been funded by the Robert Wood Johnson Foundation (RWJF) with the potential for additional funding from a competitive grant for planning and implementation. The preliminary planning proposal, originally submitted to the RWJF in 1989, was based on the recommendations of the Brieger Report, which was submitted to Dean Richard Ross in 1987. The purpose of the preliminary planning grant was to allow twelve medical schools to vie for eight $2.5-million five-year grants to implement their proposed curricula, which were to be planned during the eighteen months covered by the preliminary planning grant. That planning grant had been awarded to Johns Hopkins as of September 1, 1990, and nothing had been done because a coordinator had not yet been selected. We were already two months behind when I came to the dean's office in November 1990.

The initial phase of developing a plan for curricular change involved my doing a brief historical review of the education of medical students at Johns Hopkins, which led me to the Brieger Report, which had sat on the shelf for three years waiting for the new dean to take office. That document contained many, but not all, of the elements necessary for a curriculum of the twenty-first century. Further, because it had not been formally discussed in more than three years, many key faculty and administrators were only tangentially aware of what it contained. In addition, several key faculty were not aware of the report because they had come to Johns Hopkins within the three-year interim. This included, among others, the director of the Department of Medicine. Since the medicine department in virtually all medical schools is the largest by far of all departments, its cooperation is essential for the success of any curriculum. It therefore seemed prudent to assure solid input from that director, among others.

As presented in the Brieger Report, the goals of curricular changes were to reduce the hours spent in all basic science courses, provide at least two free afternoons each week in the first year, institute a four-year longitudinal course in clinical medicine, rearrange the schedule for preclinical courses, implement a weekly small-group discussion of topical papers to extend over the four years of medical school, provide a weekly ambulatory patient experience to span the final two years of medical school, restructure the clinical clerkships to reduce redundancy, introduce a requirement that students complete a scholarly paper, develop the teaching skills of our faculty and house staff, and improve the transition between medical school and residencies.

According to the goals of the Brieger Report, the proposed new curriculum was to include:

1. Reorientation of both preclinical and clinical instruction so that students would progress beyond the mere acquisition of facts and concepts (the vocabu-

lary and grammar of biomedical science) to a level of scientific fluency with which they could begin to think creatively about biomedical problems. Our curriculum should stimulate scientific curiosity and prepare our graduates to complete the training required to carry out original research in either a clinical or a laboratory setting.

2. Organization of the curriculum with the objective of presenting the material most logically and efficiently, and of emphasizing independent study and active learning. This would require major changes in our current schedule of required classes and electives, and enhanced coordination among courses.

3. Introduction of a four-year weekly student-faculty seminar to read and evaluate original research papers. Each seminar would consist of eight to twelve students, one basic scientist, and one physician. In the first year the students would learn how to evaluate the scientific literature critically. Advanced students would keep abreast of developments in the basic biomedical, social, and behavioral sciences and of the relevance of those developments to solving clinical problems.

4. Creation of a four-year longitudinal course that in the first two years emphasizes clinical skills, epidemiology, ethics, and the history of medicine, as well as the principles of clinical decision making, preventive medicine, and the psychosocial aspects of patient care. This course would provide the basis for an appreciation of the social and biological challenges explicit in patient care, and it would introduce students to patients from the beginning of their first year. In the final two years, the course would provide continuing ambulatory care teaching in appropriate settings.

5. The requirement that students do original research and report it in a thesis, and that time be provided in the curriculum for research and writing. The subject of the research could be in any area of basic science or clinical medicine, and could include topics in the social sciences, epidemiology, or the humanities as they pertained to medicine.

6. Restructuring of clinical clerkships to eliminate redundancies and to focus on the intellectual content of the clinical sciences. The goals of the clerkships would be reexamined, with emphasis placed on the understanding of the expected normal as well as the unexpected abnormal, clinical problem solving, and discussion of advances in each specific field. Since students would have substantial experience with ambulatory patient care in the four-year longitudinal course, the time allotted to clerkships could be reduced.

7. Appointment of a coordinator of medical education, fully empowered by the dean and the Advisory Board of the Medical Faculty to implement these recommendations, to oversee the formation of a new curriculum, and to foster improved coordination among courses.

It is interesting to note how much overlap there is between the Brieger Report and the proposal that finally was instituted.

The Educational Planning Committee

Knowing that it is essential to secure the support of key individuals if one is to have any chance of successfully altering any curriculum, the membership of the Brieger committee was reviewed, and it was noted that certain key individuals were conspicuous by their absence. Therefore, the dean named an ad hoc Educational Planning Committee (EPLC) in November 1990. The charge was to develop an outline for what a new curriculum would contain. If the result met the conditions for submission of a full grant application to the RWJF, we would do so; however, that was not to influence what the committee would plan. The committee was chaired by Dr. John Stobo, director of the Department of Medicine, who had not served on the Brieger committee. The co-chair was Dr. Thomas Pollard, director of the Department of Cell Biology and Anatomy, who had been a very active member of the Brieger committee. The rest of the committee consisted of five other clinical and basic science department directors and a resident who recently had graduated from the school of medicine. I served as the dean's staff member for the EPLC.

A few of the members suggested that the EPLC use the Brieger Report as a basis for its deliberations. However, the chair and others thought that the committee should not be constrained by the previous report or any existing curriculum structure. The idea was to assume that the Johns Hopkins University School of Medicine no longer existed! If we were to start afresh to build the medical school, what would be the optimal way to teach young persons to become outstanding physicians for the twenty-first century? Therefore, the EPLC's main contact with the Brieger Report was through the co-chair's previous involvement with the Brieger committee, the fact that some of the members had already read the full report, and the use of selected parts of the report as background information for specific discussions.

Mission Statement. The initial task of the EPLC was to determine the goals of the educational process. The curriculum itself would be the means to achieve these goals. As a first step, a mission statement was needed to guide the process. To this end, the committee was provided with copies of statements from other past committees regarding the mission of the school and the Brieger committee's "Statement of Purpose." The EPLC's final version of the mission statement differed only slightly from that suggested in the Brieger Report and by only one word from the version then in place. The final version reads: "The overall mission of the Johns Hopkins School of Medicine is to prepare physicians to practice compassionate clinical medicine of the highest standard and to identify and solve fundamental questions in the mechanisms, prevention, and treatment of disease, in health care delivery or in the basic sciences."

The only substantial alteration to our previous mission statement was to add the word *prevention.*

Goals. The next task undertaken by the EPLC was to establish specific educational goals and general methods for accomplishing them. This project involved some very lively dialogue over several months. When the dust settled, the following goals were acceptable to all members:

The highest priority of the process by which we educate physicians must be the well-being of the patients we serve. Therefore, the *goals* of the educational process must be to:

A. educate wise, intellectually curious, and compassionate physicians, ready for a lifetime of learning and problem solving aimed at furthering the well-being of the patients they serve;
B. have the flexibility to educate individuals who can serve the needs of their patients through a variety of career pathways (e.g., research, practice, development of health care policy);
C. educate individuals who are accomplished in health maintenance and disease prevention;
D. educate individuals who are prepared to address contemporary medical problems;
E. reinforce the concept that, as professionals, physicians have an obligation to function in an altruistic manner.

To accomplish these educational goals the curriculum must:

1. nurture leadership potential in whatever career pathway a student chooses, including the generation, promulgation, and/or application of medical knowledge;
2. continually foster the humanistic skills of students;
3. provide time for students to be critical thinkers;
4. require scholarly activity based on independent, creative thinking;
5. foster a mentoring relationship between student and teacher;
6. blend basic science and clinical training longitudinally instead of two years of basic science instruction followed by two years of clinical training;
7. educate students broadly, including communication and interviewing skills, critical evaluation of the medical literature, basic research methodologies, disease prevention, ethics, substance abuse, health care policy, and the economics of health care.

EPLC realized that these goals were quite general and that, in retrospect, they differed only modestly from those established by the Brieger committee. However, even though the process of determining the goals had involved much time and effort to accomplish essentially the same results, it had been necessary to ensure the support of key faculty leaders, and the fact that two separate and individual committees at two different points in time had achieved essentially the same outcome provided reassurance for inter-rater or interdeveloper reliability. Also, since these goals melded nicely with those set by the RWJF, we decided to pursue the grant.

The Educational Policy Committee

It was now the spring of 1991. The next task of the Educational Planning Committee was to develop specific objectives to further develop the process for ultimate implementation and evaluation of the curriculum. The individuals on the Educational Planning Committee were not necessarily experienced in planning a process for developing pragmatic objectives and developing implementation procedures to accomplish them. In addition, the school of medicine had had a longstanding Educational Policy Committee (EPC), which was responsible for overseeing the ongoing active curriculum. I chaired that committee, which was composed of the directors of all required courses, the associate dean of students, the director of the William H. Welch Medical Library, the registrar, and student representatives from each class. Those faculty who were most familiar with the day-to-day operations of the curriculum had expressed some confusion and concern about their role in the new curriculum, especially since the new EPLC had assumed such importance in developing the mission, goals, and objectives of the new curriculum.

This proved to be a rather delicate issue because, while it was essential to have substantial input and support from key administrative faculty (the Educational Planning Committee), the ongoing curriculum would lie in the hands of those who had spent and would spend a significant amount of time directly involved with the curriculum (the Educational Policy Committee). The resolution of the problem was for the EPLC to request that the EPC develop specific methodologies to achieve each of the seven general goals. To that end, seven subcommittees were formed within the EPLC, each of which assumed responsibility for one goal. Members of the EPC and other key faculty served on each subcommittee, which was chaired by a member of the EPC. The short-term effect was to expand the ad hoc EPLC to thirty-eight members, including representatives from all departments and six medical students. The original EPC would then carry on with their implementation and oversight of the curriculum once the expanded EPLC had issued its final report and disbanded.

Dean Michael Jones called a one-day retreat in the spring of 1991, which was attended by the directors of every department and other key faculty and staff. The overall mission statement and the educational goals approved by the EPC were reviewed and adopted by all present. The group then divided into smaller sections for further discussion and recommendations. The recommendations from the smaller sections were then combined and discussed by the large group. The items adopted by the entire group were ultimately incorporated in the final curriculum proposal.

Over the next three to four months, each of the seven subcommittees met on a number of occasions to develop at least two proposals for achieving each of the seven goals. Some of the educational goals were much more specific than others, and the subcommittees working on them had an easier task. However, all of the subcommittees met the deadline of submitting their reports by mid-July 1991. That deadline was essential because we had agreed that the goals were very much in line with those set by the RWJF for its program "Preparing Physicians for the Future: A Program in Medical Education." The deadline for that five-year grant proposal was October 1, 1991. The EPLC had agreed earlier that I could write the draft grant proposal on the basis of what we had already decided. The implementation section would be added when all of the subcommittee reports were submitted, and then a specific methodology would be selected for each goal. This proved to be very much like trying to ride a bicycle while building it, and it was essential for me to work very closely with the seven subcommittees.

One of the most interesting aspects of simultaneously working with so many different subcommittees and with the EPLC and the EPC was the incredibly different perspectives of the various members. First, with a few notable exceptions, the members of the EPLC (almost all of whom were department directors) had very little concept of exactly how much time and effort it would take to implement a fully developed specific course. Their interests were much more global, which is not surprising, since that was one of the qualities that made them good department directors. By contrast, the faculty who would be responsible for implementing proposed changes were quite reluctant to alter the status quo. They were only too aware that any change would translate into more work for them, at least at the beginning, and possible loss of control over their courses.

The key to ensuring realistic proposals for the curriculum was the interchange between these groups. The altering of our policies for promotions (discussed below), in which teaching, per se, is included as a specific requirement, is one example of a result that was essential to the successful implementation of the curriculum. Creating a sense of trust between the administration and the faculty was vital. One good way to engender that spirit is to have the various individuals work together toward a goal, especially when it involves meeting to work out specifics. When everyone has a sense of ownership and feels that he or she plays a significant role in the planning, the likelihood of successful implementation rises substantially.

The Robert Wood Johnson Foundation Grant Proposal

Between July and September 1991, the final proposal for the RWJF had to be prepared. As stated before, the dean had made a commitment to implement the new curriculum as soon as possible, with or without the funding from the RWJF. However, it soon became quite evident that having $2.5 million over five years from an outside source would move the process along significantly. This was true not only because of the money, per se, but also because of the assumption of so many of our faculty and administrators that something is inherently more valuable if someone outside the institution is willing to provide funding. In addition, having grant funding stimulated activity and progress that might not have been possible without the externally dictated time deadlines.

Writing a grant proposal required specific delineation of goals, objectives, courses, governance, faculty and staff, funding, and criteria for evaluation of the new curriculum.

Choosing the Leaders

With the basic goals having been established by the EPLC, the next step was to name, and network with, the various individuals who would translate the objectives and proposals of the expanded EPLC into courses and programs and then implement the curriculum. Among other things, the various key individuals who would assume leadership for the actual implementation of the programs had to be chosen. This was not too difficult for a number of the components, but leaders for other components would have to be chosen on the basis of their potential and experience with other projects, and other leaders would emerge only after we had implemented the curriculum. Obviously, the first-year segments had to receive primary attention, with lesser, but substantial, attention provided for the second year, and so on.

The obvious person to coordinate the initiative for the basic science component of the first year was Dr. Thomas Pollard. He had served on the Brieger committee, had co-chaired the EPLC, was director of the Department of Cell Biology and Anatomy, and was a respected researcher and educator, and a leader among the basic science directors and faculty. The outcome of his coordination and the work of many faculty is described in chapter 3.

The natural coordinator for the bridging sciences component of the second year was Dr. Langford Kidd, who had been the director of the second-year Human Pathophysiology course while serving as the chief of the Division of Pediatric Cardiology. He had decided to step down as division chief and was seeking a more active role in education. Since he had been a respected leader in the second-year curriculum, he was a natural to assume the new role. The results of his initiatives and those of almost a hundred faculty involved in the bridging sciences are described in chapter 4.

Both of these leaders immediately began to work with their constituents to develop sound programs. Each held a one-day retreat at a nearby hotel with his key faculty to begin the development of the specific courses. These retreats were followed by frequent meetings. The first-year basic science group met weekly for the better part of six months; the second-year group met less frequently because they had more time before their component was to be implemented.

Choosing the coordinator for the four-year longitudinal Physician and Society course was a challenge. Since my first year of medical school, I had viewed this kind of course as something vital that had been missing from medical education. It would take an extraordinary physician leader to understand, plan, and implement the course. While several individuals were considered capable of filling that role with great expertise, the issue of time commitment (it was to be a four-year course, after all) was a potential barrier to our enticing the correct individual. Fate again helped, in that our top choice, Dr. Leon Gordis, a highly regarded physician educator who had directed our Clinical Epidemiology course for many years and who had directed the Department of Epidemiology in the Johns Hopkins University School of Hygiene and Public Health for eighteen years, had decided to step down as director of the department. His willingness to direct the course was viewed as especially important because it would also serve to make a stronger bridge between the school of medicine and the school of hygiene and public health. Dr. Gordis already held primary appointments in both schools. He requested that Dr. Henry Seidel be named co-director of the course. This suggestion was adopted with enthusiasm. Dr. Seidel had been the associate dean of students for many years and had recently retired. He enthusiastically accepted the offer. The Physician and Society course led by Drs. Gordis and Seidel is described in chapter 5.

Finding a coordinator for the Introduction to Clinical Medicine course was very difficult. That course, which would place first-year students in the offices of private practicing physicians from the community, had not been enthusiastically embraced by a few of the members of the EPC. One outspoken member felt especially strongly that it would be a waste of time. The school had attempted something similar years earlier, and it had not been at all successful. However, that program had provided a brief clinical experience lasting one quarter and had been meant to augment the Introduction to Clinical Skills course. Apparently the oversight had not been good, and the quality of the teaching had been varied. The fact that a previous similar program had failed made the choice of a director especially important if the course was to succeed. Since none of the community-based part-time faculty had been involved in directing anything like this program, I decided to coordinate it personally for a year and to allow the ultimate director to emerge from among the physicians who would precept the students in their offices. That proved to be a sound plan, and after the first year it became obvious that Dr. Richard Freeman would be that leader. Like all the other physician preceptors for that course, Dr. Freeman had a part-time faculty appointment in the school of medicine. He accepted the challenge of directing the program (beginning with the second iteration) with great enthusiasm. The result is discussed in chapter 7.

Another important person to be named was someone who would provide leadership as a nonphysician medical educator. Amazingly, the Johns Hopkins University School of Medicine had never had such a person, much less an office for medical education. It was clear that we needed someone with expertise who could assist our faculty in the design, implementation, and evaluation of various courses. Because many of our faculty members were unaccustomed to working with such an individual, it was essential to choose a very mature person who had expertise and an easygoing personality. I had begun a national search for such an individual in the spring, and it resulted in the hiring of Dr. John Shatzer in October 1991. The successful results of his leadership and interactions with a variety of faculty are discussed in chapter 9.

The final key individual to be named was someone who would lead the initiatives with computers and in medical informatics. There didn't appear to be anyone on the faculty or staff with exactly the right qualifications, and I feared that we might not be able to find a leader before we were well into the planning and implementation of the first courses. Fortunately I was incorrect. Dr. Harold Lehmann, a pediatrician who had been one of my fellows in General Academic Pediatrics at Johns Hopkins, had gone on to receive a Ph.D. in medical informatics at Stanford University. He had come to visit me to discuss his potential employment at various medical institutions around the country. In what can be described as a "eureka" moment by some (or a "duh" moment by others), it occurred to me that Harold just might fulfill our needs. I described what I had in mind, he greatly expanded those ideas, and I hired him. He joined our faculty in January 1993 and over the course of several years has taken the program far beyond what any of us imagined. This process is described in chapter 6.

Since there was time to plan for the third and fourth years, choosing leaders for those later courses was delayed until the EPC had had more time to decide what should be done in those years. At this point, we became very engaged in planning for the site visit by the RWJF team who would decide if we were to be one of the eight programs to receive the coveted grant.

The Site Visit

Nothing can generate more productive, coordinated activity in academic centers than an upcoming site visit for a grant. In late October 1991, we were notified that we were to be site-visited in mid-December 1991. Within those six weeks, we were able to formulate more-or-less specific plans for the implementation of the curriculum. The first year of the curriculum was fairly well developed, and we believed that it could be implemented by the following September (1992). The second year was less well developed but had sufficient specificity that we were confident that it could be implemented by September 1993. The last two years of the curriculum were even less well developed, but plans for their implementation were well outlined. Some of the site visitors doubted that we could, indeed, implement the first year in less than nine months. This skepticism stimulated our faculty to accept the challenge with greater enthusiasm and to state this with great confidence at the site visit. The site visitors must have been convinced, because we were informed in mid-February that we would receive the grant funding, which would be forthcoming beginning on March 1, 1992.

I should add that we also had been site-visited by the Liaison Committee on Medical Education for our accreditation in December 1992. That team was so doubtful about our ability to fully implement the new curriculum that they required a written update in two years. Their doubtfulness fired the enthusiasm of our faculty even more, and we took great delight in sending the written report of our success two years later.

My reason for emphasizing the role of outsiders' doubt is to point out how good faculty, who believe in themselves and their co-workers, can respond to challenge. A vital force is engaged when faculty support each other and receive support from the administration. I feel sure that we would not have been able to plan and implement the entire new curriculum in the relatively short time of five years without outside support, but we would have been able to do it over a longer period of time, although the programs that required new monies, such as the Physician and Society course and the Office of Medical Informatics Education, would have been implemented later.

The Proposed Curriculum

Our curriculum, as planned and implemented, has seven basic goals:

1. the integration of basic science and clinical experiences;
2. expanded use of case-based, small-group learning sessions;

3. early experience with community-based practicing physicians;
4. development of a four-year longitudinal Physician and Society course to teach students that medicine does not exist in a social vacuum (this course involves ethics; fine arts such as music, literature, and painting as they relate to medicine; legal issues; finances; political issues; history of medicine; and so on);
5. computerization of learning and teaching, to educate our students to use electronic networks and databases effectively for patient care and research;
6. expanded experiences in ambulatory settings in the required clinical courses; and
7. rewarding faculty for teaching.

These goals were achieved by

1. altering all four years of our curriculum to ensure the integration of basic science and clinical experiences (goal 1), making expanded use of case-based, small-group learning sessions (goal 2), and offering expanded experiences in ambulatory settings in the required clinical courses (goal 6);
2. developing an experience in the offices of community-based private-practice physicians that would extend through the entire first year (goal 3);
3. developing a Physician and Society course that would extend for all four years of medical school (goal 4);
4. funding and employing the full services of a physician-led team with expertise in medical informatics and the use of computers in medicine (goal 5);
5. changing the policies and procedures for advancement to specifically reward faculty for teaching (goal 7);
6. providing additional financial remuneration for faculty involved in small-group and ambulatory clinical teaching settings (goal 7);
7. developing a special medical education center with large and small conference rooms, patient-centered examination rooms equipped with audio-visual facilities, and a section for computer learning; and
8. evaluating, to the extent that we can, the effects of the curricular changes.

These goals and methods of achievement formed the basis for all work on the curriculum over the next five years. The first year (1991/92) was devoted to specific course design for the first-year courses, including all of the basic science courses (chap. 3), the first year of the Physician and Society course (chap. 5), and the Introduction to Clinical Medicine course (chap. 7). The first class to matriculate under the new curriculum entered in September 1992, and all of the first-year courses had to be completely developed and ready for the students by that time.

We had more time to develop the courses to be taught in the second, third, and fourth years, but much planning for all years occurred during 1991/92. It is important to remember that the faculty for all four years had to develop the new courses while still teaching their ongoing classes according to the "old curriculum."

The First-Year Curriculum

It was imperative for those who would be responsible for the first-year courses to develop a schedule for the first year by the summer of 1992. Ultimately, the first year's weekly schedule was as shown in table 2.1.

During the planning year, the faculty and students had agreed that the major problems with the old curriculum were that the class days were too long and that the courses were too dense and contained too many lectures. Many faculty members believed that this resulted in students' barely reading anything except the

Table 2.1 First-Year Weekly Schedule

Time	Monday	Tuesday	Wednesday	Thursday	Friday
8:00 A.M.	Lecture	Lecture	Lecture	Lecture	Lecture
9:15 A.M.	Discussion/ lab[a]	Journal club[b]	Discussion/ lab	Discussion/ lab	Discussion/ lab
10:30 A.M.		Discussion/			
11:00 A.M.		lab	PAS[c]		
12:00 noon	Lecture	Lecture	PAS	Lecture	Lecture
2:00 P.M.					Clinical Correlations[d]

Note: One afternoon session every other week was spent with a community-based physician on either Monday, Tuesday, or Wednesday afternoon.

[a]Discussion/lab: small-group discussion of problem sets, or lab taught to group of fifteen students.

[b]Journal club: a weekly meeting of groups of fifteen students at which a paper is read from the current literature relevant to the students' current courses. The students discuss the paper with a junior faculty member from a clinical departmrent and rotating faculty from the basic science departments (two faculty per session).

[c]PAS: Physician and Society course.

[d]Clinical Correlations: a Friday clinic involving a patient presentation, an analysis of clinical features, and a strong basic science component designed to integrate the main concepts covered during the week.

Table 2.2   First-Year Total Hours

	Curriculum	
	Old	New
Lectures	19	10
Labs	12	12
Clinical experience	0	4
Small groups	1	3
Total	32	29

handouts and assigned sections of textbooks. This feeling was given some credibility by a study involving medical students at the University of Southern California.[1] Therefore, the first-year faculty agreed to change the seven-hour schedule (9 A.M. to 5 P.M. with an hour off for lunch) to a five-hour schedule (8 A.M. to 1 P.M.). The idea was to allow students to have unscheduled time almost every afternoon for self-guided learning—reading, using the computer-based education facilities, or studying with their colleagues.

To make up for the lost hours, classes were extended by three weeks, so that students did not complete the first year until mid-June. Surprisingly, we encountered no problems with this. The students felt that it was worth the extra three weeks in order to have a decompressed first year in which they didn't feel as though they were on a treadmill. During the first three years of the new curriculum, I met with groups of students when they returned from the winter holidays. The recurring theme was the perceived differences in their own stress levels compared with those of their friends at other medical schools that had traditional lecture-intense first-year schedules.

Another aspect of the first year was that most faculty and students were satisfied with the switch away from lectures to small groups. When the new, extended-year schedule was compared with the previous schedule, there was a marked difference in the type of teaching but not much in total hours. This is shown in table 2.2.

The Introduction to Clinical Medicine Course

While the basic science course directors and the Physician and Society group were working on their respective courses, a program in which every first-year medical student would spend time with community-based physicians needed to be developed. The major task was to find a sufficient number of physicians who would be willing to take students into their busy practices. This was not going to be easy, for a number of reasons. First of all, the students would be totally inexperienced, since this program was to begin during the first week of class. Second, the pressures of managed care made it more difficult than ever for private practitioners to spend time with students. Third, we had no way to reimburse the clinicians financially.

We were adamant that the goal of the program was not to teach clinical skills but to socialize the students to what it means to be a physician. However, even having the students serving in an observer role took extra time, because the patients, office staff, and students had to be oriented; in addition, some patients might object to having a medical student present.

It is important to note that Johns Hopkins has a one-track system for promotion. Community-based physicians who participate in the medical school are provided with part-time faculty appointments, mostly without financial reimbursement. Unlike full-time faculty, these part-time faculty members are not bound by the requirement that individuals spend only a limited time in each faculty rank before a decision must be made for promotion or termination of contract. In general, the requirement for receiving and keeping these part-time appointments is participation in the education and training of medical students, residents, fellows, or graduate students. As might be expected, the physicians we were to contact were those who were already heavily involved in teaching.

Because it was going to take some persuasion to enlist sufficient physicians, I decided to personally call every potential mentor. I enlisted the assistance of Dr. Franklin Herlong, the associate dean of medical student affairs, and Dr. Henry Seidel, the former associate dean of students, who had served in that capacity for thirteen years. Each of them provided me with a list of community-based physicians who would be excellent role models. In some cases, in which they had a close personal relationship with the physician, they called him or her personally, and I followed up with another call soon thereafter. In all cases, I called the physician to solicit his or her help. The three of us together developed a list of about eighty potential mentors.

Because I wanted this program to be sufficiently flexible, the only thing I told each potential mentor was that the students were to be with them beginning in the first week of their first year and that none had any professional experience with physicians. The goal was to provide the students with a general experience of how a physician in private practice functions and to allow them to interact in a general role with patients. We would have several meetings during the year, the first to be held a few weeks before September 1992, in which the mentors would be oriented to what was expected. I told them that the program would be an opportunity for them to have a profound impact on the early education of medical students and that all of their suggestions would be taken seriously.

To my amazement, only one of the first sixty-two physicians I called said that he would not be able to participate. One hundred twenty-three students were due to matriculate, and each physician was asked to take two students, each of whom would be at the office one afternoon every other week. That meant that one student would be present in each physician's office for one afternoon each week.

Because many of the offices were not within walking distance of the medical school and were outside the area covered by our shuttle-bus system, we had to determine which students had cars. We sent each student a mail-back card on which to provide us that information before matriculation. It was the first and only time we would achieve an astounding 100 percent response rate from medical students on the first attempt. As it turned out, plans had to be revised when the students actually began their experiences, because some who had thought that they would have a car didn't, and some who hadn't anticipated having a car did. That was one of many necessary adjustments.

From that modest beginning, a very popular and effective course developed over the years, as the directorship was handed over to a community-based faculty member. The process through which that success was achieved is described in detail in chapter 7.

The Clinical Epidemiology Course

Clinical Epidemiology had been taught in the second year, but the decision was made to move it into the first year to prepare students for the weekly journal clubs that were to be a component of the basic science courses. Moving Clinical Epidemiology from the second to the first year was not going to be easy. It would mean that the course director and faculty would have to teach the course twice in the first year of implementation—that is, teaching the second-year students in the traditional curriculum and the first-year students in the new curriculum. To further complicate matters, several of those who taught this course were faculty from the Johns Hopkins University School of Hygiene and Public Health. To complete the potential logistic nightmare, the course director was Dr. Gordis, who also had agreed to direct the Physician and Society course. There is no greater example of goodwill and desire to be team players than the cooperation shown by Dr. Gordis and the faculty who agreed to allow the switch.

After one year, the feedback from students and the basic science faculty stimulated the course director to add a component of basic biostatistics to the course. This was the only significant content alteration made to a course that had always been very popular and effective with the students. However, another course director was named after two years because Dr. Gordis had become too involved in his other responsibilities, including his role as director of the Physician and Society course.

The Physician and Society Course

History of Medicine and Ethics had been taught as two short courses in the first year. Ethics was to be the underlying theme of the new Physician and Society course, and History of Medicine was to be integrated into the first year of that course. The details for those segments were left up to Dr. Gordis, the director of the new course, and his group.

Actually, the more appropriate title for this course would have been Physician *in* Society, but when I was writing the grant proposal, I realized that the initials lent themselves to potential mischief by the students. To eliminate that possibility for what was one of the most innovative components of the curriculum, the title was changed to Physician *and* Society.

Since this was a completely new course that would span all four years of the curriculum, it required a tremendous amount of time and energy on the part of almost a hundred faculty. The details involved in the planning and implementation of this course—or actually, courses—are described in chapter 5.

The Second-Year Curriculum

While the first-year course directors and faculty were working on their courses and schedule, the second-year group began working on their courses and schedule. The traditional curriculum had included four major courses—Human Pathophysiology, Pathology, Pharmacology, and Clinical Skills—that spanned the first three quarters of the second year. The fourth quarter marked the beginning of the clinical rotations, which were the responsibility of other faculty. In addition, two other courses—short courses in Clinical Epidemiology and the History of Medicine—had been taught in the first quarter of the second year.

It was essential to have a great deal of integration between the first- and second-year courses and agreement among the various course directors. Since the first-year curriculum was to be reduced somewhat in hours and to have courses that began with normal cells and ended with normal systems, it seemed logical for the second year to continue with organ-systems-based teaching. Further, some of the material traditionally taught in the first year fit better into the second, and vice versa. The easiest way to accomplish these changes would have been for the leaders of the first and the second years to meet on a regular basis and agree on the final placement of courses and material to be taught. In actuality, such meetings occurred only a few times, and most of the agreements were negotiated by my acting as an intermediary. The members of the first-year committee were under great pressure to develop their courses and schedule while simultaneously teaching students the traditional curriculum. There simply was not sufficient time for them to meet with the second-year group, who also were working very hard but had one more year than the first-year group to develop their courses.

Items for which there had to be negotiated agreements included the second year's being taught by organ systems and the movement of the topic of Behavior from the first year to the second year. Behavior had been taught as part of the first-year course in Neurology, which would now be taught in the Neuroscience section of systems in the first year. Teaching by systems was relatively easily negotiated. No one had significant objections to the concept, including those who believed that it made no difference how we taught the courses so long as the students were smart and the faculty were good teachers. The details of how the systems concept would be introduced were left to the second-year coordinator and course directors.

That left the issue of where the Behavior section was to fit in the curriculum. It seemed most logical that it would be part of a Neurology and Behavior segment of the second year. The major problem was that this course was taught by members of the Department of Psychiatry, and they had fit it into their schedules as a course for first-year students. As it turned out, after several meetings with the course director and the department director, the section was moved to the second year. This allowed the faculty to have a year in which they taught no course (since it would be moved to the second year), allowing them additional time to prepare to teach the course to second-year students as part of systems. Ironically, after this schedule was tried for four years, we decided to move most of the Behavior section back to the first year to decompress the second year. Again, the goodwill and cooperation of the department director, Dr. Paul McHugh, and the course director, Dr. Peter Rabins, were essential to accomplish this change.

While these logistic maneuvers were being negotiated, Dr. Langford Kidd and the second-year committee were busy working on the specific schedule and segments for the entire second year, except for the Physician and Society course. Like the first-year group, they agreed to limit the number of lecture hours to a minimum, to integrate more small-group teaching, and (as much as possible) to reserve afternoons for clinical experiences. Because of the amount of material to be covered, even after limiting the number of hours allowed for each topic, it was not possible to allow every afternoon to be unscheduled, even in the first quarter, when only one afternoon each week was needed for the Clinical Skills course. By the third quarter, almost the entire day was filled with classes, with the afternoons filled with Clinical Skills.

One of the results of the great discrepancy in daily class hours between the first and second years was that many members of the index class were quite stressed several weeks into the second year. Some of the faculty felt that it was probably a delayed reaction to the reality of medical school. Others felt that some of the material taught in the second year should be moved back into the first year or that the second year should be extended into the fourth quarter. Both of these suggestions were debated extensively by the EPC, and it was decided not to change. The first year had been a success, and it seemed too soon to make any significant alterations. Also, the students did not want to give up the extra quarter of clinical time; they told us that they would rather have a relatively compressed second year than give up the clinical time.

For some unknown reason, since no significant alteration had been made in class time, the second class that was exposed to the new curriculum (and all subsequent classes) had no major complaints about the density of the second-year courses. One theory to explain this phenomenon is that the index class had complained so intensely to the class behind them that the reality of the situation never lived up to what the subsequent class had expected. In any case, the situation became a nonproblem. Nevertheless, we knew that there might be some decompression in the second-year curriculum as we progressed in the process, because we wanted to reduce the substantial discrepancy in density between years. Indeed, that is what happened when approximately fifty hours of the Behavior section were moved back into the first year, using a few afternoons each week. This occurred in the third and fourth modules, in keeping with the students' feeling that unscheduled afternoons were most advantageous when they occurred in the first and second modules.

While all of this was going on, Dr. Kidd and his course directors were working with more than eighty faculty members who were involved in teaching the second-year Pathology, Human Pathophysiology, and Pharmacology courses. What finally evolved is described in detail in chapter 4.

When all of the courses are included, the basic second-year schedule finally agreed upon by all course directors was as shown in table 2.3. Like the first-year planning group, the second-year group also accomplished a marked change in the number of hours devoted to lectures and labs and the number of hours devoted to small groups. The second-year course hours are shown in table 2.4.

The Third- and Fourth-Year Curricula

Even though it would be almost three years before any changes were incorporated into the third and fourth years for the clinical rotations or for any other courses we had initiated, we knew that it would take a great deal of time to decide what to do and how to do it. Therefore, planning for the third and fourth years began at the same time as planning for the first and second years. Because of the complexity involved in changing clinical rotations and the number of fac-

Table 2.3   Second-Year Weekly Schedule

Time	Monday	Tuesday	Wednesday	Thursday	Friday
Quarters 1 and 2					
8 A.M.–1 P.M.	Core[a]	Core	Core	Core	Core
2 P.M.–5 P.M.	Clinical Skills/IS[c]	PAS[b]	Clinical Skills/IS	IS[c]	IS
Quarter 3					
8 A.M.–1 P.M.	Core	Core	Core	Core	Core
2 P.M.–5 P.M.	Clinical Skills	PAS	Clinical Skills	Clinical Skills	IS

[a]Core = Pathology, Human Pathophysiology, and Pharmacology.
[b]PAS = Physician and Society course.
[c]IS = Independent study time.

ulty who were already involved or who would be involved, the EPC meetings were to be the forum for discussions, and the EPC was to be the ultimate decision maker for the last quarter of the second year and the third and fourth years of the curriculum.

We began by asking each of the directors of the current required clinical courses to prepare a brief written document and to make a formal presentation of his or her current rotation at one of the EPC meetings. The directors were also to describe any changes that they thought would lead to a better experience for the students and to outline what would be needed to implement such changes. This was to include potential changes in the amount of time students would spend on the rotation. One rotation was presented at each of the monthly EPC meetings. It took almost two years to complete this process because other issues pertaining to the first- or second-year courses needed to be discussed intermittently.

Table 2.4   Second-Year Total Hours

	Curriculum	
	Old	New
Lectures	18	14
Labs	18	8
Clinical skills	4–12	4–12
Small groups	0	14
Total	40–48	40–48

In September 1992, a pilot program had been initiated to provide a few third-year students with longitudinal patient experiences. Five general internists and pediatricians from the full-time faculty volunteered to have one student join each of them in their clinics one afternoon a week for a year to follow a panel of patients. A few students—mostly those who were spending a year working on a research project or obtaining a master's degree in public health—had had such experiences in the past on an ad hoc basis with various faculty members. The longitudinal patient experiences reportedly were successful, but we wanted to monitor a specific pilot program to decide if they might serve as a model for general, outpatient experiences for all students. After two years, it was decided that another mechanism would be more reasonable because of the numbers of students involved and the intensity of input required of the faculty. However, these experiences remain as popular electives for a few students each year.

In May 1993, the dean held a retreat on the medical curriculum. The attendees included the provost, all senior members of the dean's office, the president of the Johns Hopkins Hospital, all department directors, and all key faculty members involved in the planning and implementation of the new curriculum. After presentations about the curriculum in general, and lengthy discussions about promoting generalism and primary care in the curriculum, the group directed the EPC to develop sufficient general medical experiences (on and off site) as required rotations for all students. The biggest problem was to develop a program for ambulatory general internal medicine. The old nine-week rotation in medicine contained no required ambulatory general internal medicine experiences. A subcommittee of the EPC was assigned the task of developing a plan for a program in generalism. In the meantime, the EPC worked on other plans for the general medical experience for students. At the September 1993 EPC meeting, a subcommittee was appointed to develop a proposal for a generalist clerkship. This committee completed its report by February 1994. This is described in chapter 8.

By May 1994, each clinical course director had presented his or her clinical clerkship. A retreat of EPC members and several other key faculty was held in July 1994 to discuss the generalism proposal and to decide exactly what changes were to be made regarding the time allotted for each clinical clerkship. The exact curriculum for each clerkship was left up to the appropriate department. The only specific guideline was that at least 25 percent of the time spent in every clerkship was to be in the ambulatory setting. The specifics of what evolved for the generalism clerkship and all of the required clinical clerkships are described in chapter 8.

One final issue to be resolved was how to reintegrate the basic sciences into the third and fourth years. The planning for this reintegration was not initiated to any degree until we were a full year into the implemented curriculum. Because there are only so many hours in one day and there is a limit to what can be asked of any faculty, no matter how enthusiastic and cooperative, I assumed the responsibility for developing a plan for this aspect of the curriculum. By the time this planning was initiated, a director for Introduction to Clinical Medicine had been found, and I no longer had direct responsibility for that course. Further, the planning would not involve increased teaching time for anyone, so I could proceed without compromising the goodwill of the faculty. The first step was to send a very brief survey to each of the basic science department directors asking if they had any ideas for or interest in reintroducing basic science into the third and fourth years. The responses were surprisingly positive, and several ideas evolved into the plan for the clinical years that is described in chapter 3.

The Office of Medical Education Services

When Dr. Shatzer, director of medical education services, began work in October 1992, he offered his assistance to any of the course directors or faculty who were developing specific courses. His original offer was met with various degrees of enthusiasm. Most of the basic scientists were not certain of what he might add. I believe that they were so involved with getting themselves to agree on a unified, nondepartmentally based curriculum that they did not consider the addition of an "outsider" favorably. In fact, it was clear that they viewed my own presence at their meetings as potential interference from the dean's office. It was important to respect their desire to develop their area of expertise with no more oversight from the dean's office than was needed to assure a coordinated curriculum. Fortunately, Dr. Shatzer and I had discussed this before he came to Johns Hopkins, and he was comfortable with waiting, and gaining their confidence over time.

In the meantime, his input was welcomed by those working with other aspects of the curriculum. He attended many of the planning meetings of the Introduction to Clinical Medicine course, the Physician and Society course, and the second-year planning committee. He offered a perspective not generally known to our physician educators. In addition, within months of his arrival and the arrival of Dr. Lehmann, we began to plan for a Clinical Education Center.

One of the frustrations of the clinical course directors was the lack of designated clinical teaching space. In addition, Dr. Shatzer expressed a need for a number of rooms that could serve as mock examining rooms and in which audiovideo cameras could be mounted. A monitor room, where faculty preceptors could work either alone or with the students to evaluate the students' performances on the videos, was also needed. Dr. Shatzer had planned to initiate a program to augment clinical teaching using standardized patients, and this type of teaching and learning space was vital. In addition, we needed a designated space for the students' educational clinical experiences that was separate from the hospital-, clinic-, and office-based spaces where students currently interacted with patients.

After a great deal of negotiating, we were able to obtain space for a Clinical Education Center that would be located in the Johns Hopkins Hospital rather than in the medical school buildings. In July 1992, the Women's Board of the Johns Hopkins Hospital provided a gift of $48,000 for the renovation of the space and for furniture. That center, opened in the fall of 1993, houses two suites—one for the Office of Medical Education Services, including nine examination rooms, the monitor room, and two small conference rooms; and one for the Office of Medical Informatics Education. The suite for the Office of Medical Informatics Education contains space for the development of software to be used in the curriculum. The evolution of the Clinical Education Center is discussed in chapter 8.

Dr. Shatzer also took the lead in working with a group of second- and third-year medical students to provide specific feedback and opinions on proposed new courses. Two of the students, with the assistance of Dr. Shatzer, wrote a report and formally presented it at a meeting of the first-year curriculum working group. This type of feedback was incorporated into the curriculum and occurs each year, with the dean's office providing lunch for those who attend the meeting. A number of subtle but important alterations to the courses resulted from this feedback.

Over the years, Dr. Shatzer's role in the implementation and evaluation of the curriculum has evolved, and his expertise is now sought at some level by almost every course director. A more complete discussion of the evaluation initiative is discussed in chapter 9.

The Office of Medical Informatics Education

When Dr. Lehmann arrived in January 1992, he began working with some of the planning groups to determine what role computerized information might play in specific aspects of the curriculum. His input, like Dr. Shatzer's, was accepted with various degrees of enthusiasm by different course directors and faculty members. In general, the same persons who had accepted advice from Dr. Shatzer were open to consultation with Dr. Lehmann. Dr. Lehmann had also been forewarned about the types of receptions that he would experience. However, as a physician, his expectations were higher than Dr. Shatzer's, and he was more disappointed that not all faculty members were anxious to accept his expertise. It didn't take very long for him to realize that there were many projects that needed his attention, and he wisely expended his energy on those that involved faculty who were eager for his input.

By September 1992, Dr. Lehmann had hired a programmer and an administrative assistant and developed an Office of Medical Informatics Education. Over time the value of this resource became evident, and it was to have a very profound effect on the new curriculum. The details of this work are discussed in chapter 6.

Governance

The Role of the Dean's Office

One of the major issues that was vital to the success of implementing the new curriculum was governance. While it should be obvious that a curriculum will not be initiated or changed without having a single overall coordinator who takes on the project with great enthusiasm and energy and the authority to make it happen, that concept is not necessarily accepted by all who are involved in the process. In our case, the dean had to decide that a new curriculum was a top-priority item and to delegate the administrative responsibility and authority to someone who would assure the successful completion of the project. The first part was not difficult, because the dean was a strong advocate of excellence in education, and almost everyone who thought about the curriculum believed that it could be improved. Further, a number of ad hoc committees had reported that revision of the curriculum was necessary. Even the skeptics who thought that the curriculum, per se, made little difference when good faculty and students were involved admitted that periodic major change stimulated vigor and renewed interest on the part of the faculty and administration. In addition, major change meant an influx of funds, which would provide for greater interest in teaching.

The problem was that, for the most part, responsibility for the curriculum had always been the realm of the department directors. In fact, that single issue had been primarily responsible for a rather disjointed approach to content design and method of teaching. That is, all of the key players from all departments did not plan the overall curriculum together; in many cases, the planning was done by several groups who didn't work closely with one another. As a pediatrician, I viewed some groups as still functioning at the parallel-play stage and only later advancing to the interactive-play stage of development. What really mattered was that we needed a coordinated curriculum with an overall theme, little duplication, and no omissions. To accomplish this, it was vital to have a single coordinator based in the dean's office. At various times that role involved being a visionary, mediator, target, coach, or cheerleader.

It was not going to be easy to convince department and course directors that what they had been doing for years, with obvious success, should be changed. It would also be difficult to develop a curriculum that would de-emphasize the "efficiency" of the lecture and replace lectures with small groups that required much more faculty time and preparation. The difficulty was exacerbated by the fact that research funding was becoming much more difficult to obtain and managed care was eroding the school's clinical revenues; both of these factors meant that more faculty time was needed to make up for the real or potential financial losses to the departments. Finally, it would take much convincing for the directors to give up their autonomy and authority. The more closely they were tied to the educational process, the more difficulty was anticipated.

Every success story has heroes, and some of the major heroes of this story are department directors. I am convinced that it would have taken much longer to achieve the major alteration of the first-year basic science curriculum without the strong leadership of Dr. Thomas Pollard. He had been a champion of education and took the lead in convincing the basic scientists to make the necessary changes.

In truth, he was openly cautious about the role of the dean's office in altering the basic science curriculum. Some of his caution may have been to preserve the independent image of the directors, which was essential to ensure their cooperation. Also, he was displaying feelings that probably were shared by most of the basic science faculty. It would take a while for him and most others to trust that I was not going to "take over," which would have been disastrous and foolish. One example of how Dr. Pollard was able to maintain the independence of the basic scientists while not degrading my role is as follows: Very early in the process, he accepted my offer to financially support a retreat for key basic science faculty. He politely made it clear that while Dr. Shatzer (whose input I also offered) and I were welcome to speak with the group for a short while, the meeting was to be for the basic scientists. I accepted their invitation; at the meeting I made a few brief remarks and introduced Dr. Shatzer, and then we both left the basic scientists to "do their thing." I'm not certain exactly what happened at that meeting, but the results solidified the process that was to ensure the change of the basic science curriculum. Because that was the primary purpose of the retreat, we all considered it a great success.

After this meeting, I made an effort to speak with the key basic science faculty whenever I had the opportunity, so that we could get to know one another better. It took a while, but gradually they began to understand that I was also a faculty member whose interest was the overall education of medical students. The point was eventually reached where they understood my metaphor that they were the concert musicians and I was the conductor. They played the music, and I made sure that everyone was playing from the same score. We all wanted to have a great symphony, and both components were necessary.

It took a little longer for a few of the basic science department directors to understand my role. About one year into the grant, a few of them went to the dean and complained that they didn't know how I was using the grant money. They couldn't understand why I had hired a "computer person" and a medical educator and had not used that money for the increased faculty time the new curriculum demanded. At first I was upset because they had not spoken to me but had gone directly to the dean, who had given me the authority to manage the budget. I spoke to several of the other basic science directors with whom I had by now established a very good working relationship and who had been involved in the allocation of faculty funds, and they assured me that they would support me. The few directors who had gone to the dean had not been involved as intimately with the curriculum process (by their own choice), and therefore had relatively little idea about the overall plan or the budget as a whole. I was not surprised by their questions; I did question their method of trying to get answers.

The dean and I met with them subsequently, and when I explained to them how and why the money had been allocated, they seemed to be mollified. I believe that several of the other directors had spoken with them in the interim. What started out as a negative experience turned out to be a real turning point in my relationship (and therefore the relationship of the dean's office) with the basic science directors and faculty with regard to the curriculum. Over the years, these relationships have become integrated so that careful monitoring of programs by the dean's office occurs without the loss of the faculty autonomy that breeds excellence. That delicate balance is difficult to achieve and maintain, but it is also one of the most important things necessary for a successful curriculum.

A close working relationship with the clinical department and course directors was a little easier to achieve, because I am a clinician and clinical researcher. I had a much better grasp of how the clinical departments and the clinical faculty functioned, and of the educational content of the clinical components of the curriculum. Also, I had worked more closely with many of the clinical faculty in a variety of settings before coming to the dean's office. However, the issues of departmental authority and autonomy from the dean's office were also prevalent in the clinical departments.

I had not realized the level of ambivalence with which many faculty viewed the dean's office. On the one hand, they understood and respected the authority of the dean and his designees, but on the other, they resented any loss of autonomy. Some were far removed from the decision-making aspects of the dean's office and had little or no understanding of what happened there. The only time they became aware of issues was when they personally were involved in the decisions or the outcomes of decisions. This lapse in communication occurred despite the active role of the Medical School Council as liaison between the faculty and administration (the council is composed of faculty members elected by their peers) and the link that the department directors provided between the dean's office and the faculty in their departments. Because of this, it was imperative for us to include as many individual faculty members as possible in the decision making for their courses, and for me to be as visible and available as possible to help with communication. This took a tremendous amount of time and repetition, and sometimes I was tempted to eliminate some of the meetings, but I'm very happy that I almost never did that.

In addition, the dean periodically discussed the curriculum in various settings to emphasize his support. The extra attention made a great deal of difference in what we were able to accomplish and in the attitude of the faculty. Sound communication remains the key to successful changes, no matter what they entail.

Changing Policies for Faculty Promotion

One of our stated objectives was to change the policies and procedures for academic advancement specifically to reward the faculty for teaching. Because it would take a long time to develop these policies and have them implemented, I began working with the Medical School Council very early in 1991 to develop a specific proposal for a promotion policy that rewarded teaching efforts of the faculty. This was especially important because Johns Hopkins has a one-track system for appointment and promotion, and traditional research productivity and publications were the easiest promotion criteria to identify objectively.

In 1980, a subcommittee of the Medical School Council had developed a written document for policies governing appointments, promotions, and professional activities of the full-time faculty; this document came to be known as "the Gold Book." The document was approved by the Advisory Board of the Medical Faculty, which is composed of all department directors and several other key faculty, including the chair and co-chair of the Medical School Council. Subsequently, all changes to the Gold Book required the approval of the advisory board, with full and active participation of the Medical School Council. It therefore seemed sensible to begin discussing changes with the Medical School Council.

One of my activities as associate dean and subsequently as vice dean for academic affairs and faculty was to communicate to the council, at their monthly meetings, the activities of the dean's office. It was therefore relatively easy to work with the council, especially on this project, which they strongly supported. The chair of the Medical School Council appointed a subcommittee, and it developed a policy that became the official school policy governing appointments, promotions, and professional activities of the full-time faculty in March 1992. The 1992 policy differed from its 1980 predecessor in that it more specifically designated teaching as one important form of scholarship necessary for promotion. The 1980 policy read as follows:

It is crucial to the academic health of this institution that high standards for promotion be maintained. Candidates proposed for promotion must satisfy as a first prerequisite the basic obligations specified in Article I-C. The most important criteria for promotion follow:

1. *Scholarship:* The primary basis for academic advancement is creative scholarship, defined as the substantive contribution in the areas of basic and/or clinical science. Such scholarship can influence the thought or work of others only if it is communicated or demonstrated in a form that can be passed on to peers in a given field of study, particularly in precise and effective written form. A given number of published communications is not by itself sufficient; the essence of creative scholarship in significance and quality is assessed by peer judgment.

2. *Teaching:* Close in importance to achievement in creative scholarship is excellence in teaching, whether in the lecture hall, in the conference room, at the laboratory bench, or at the bedside. Excellence in teaching connotes an objective, up-to-date, accurate, and balanced command of the field being taught, effectiveness in communicating its essence, and the willingness to interact and exchange views with students at the highest levels of intellectual integrity. Excellence in teaching connotes also intangible elements of intellectual stimulation and, indeed, inspiration. The judgments of students, trainees, and peers are important in evaluating teaching ability.

3. *Clinical Ability:* A third criterion is excellence in discharging clinical obligations, for those members of the faculty having such responsibilities. Because of the basic importance of the faculty member–clinician as a model in teaching students the practice of medicine, the professional competence, integrity, and empathy of a faculty member in teaching patients, his national or international reputation as a consultant, and his election to medical societies relevant to achievement in his field constitute important criteria for promotion.

4. *Service:* In addition to the above principal criteria for promotion, service to the Institution, as defined in Article I-C, 4, shall be an additional criterion for promotion.

The 1992 changes redefined *scholarship* and more clearly defined the importance of teaching for advancement. Subsequently, a number of faculty were promoted primarily because of their teaching excellence. However, many faculty and the Medical School Council thought that the policy could be further refined. Therefore, the policy was further changed in 1996 to more specifically define what constituted scholarship in each of the categories. That policy now reads as follows:

> The criteria for appointment and promotion are derived from the Institution's primary aim, which is to be a national and international leader in medicine, science, and education. This aim can be achieved only if the school's faculty are national and international leaders in their respective fields.
>
> Professional recognition as a leader in one's field is the fundamental criterion for promotion to the rank of professor. However, earlier in the promotional sequence, well before candidacy for professor, the prime consideration is whether a faculty member's professional career is developing in a manner that promises to make him or her eligible for promotion to the next level within the prescribed time frame. At all stages of the promotional sequence, candidates proposed for promotion must satisfy as a first prerequisite the basic obligations specified above in Article I-D, "Obligations of Full-time Faculty Members to the School of Medicine." Likewise, at all stages, the criteria for academic advancement are research, teaching, and clinical distinction, documented by meritorious publications.
>
> *Scholarship:* Scholarship, the primary basis for academic advancement, encompasses two important elements: the generation of new knowledge and the dissemination of that knowledge to others. Customarily, such new knowledge is disseminated through publication in peer-reviewed journals and books. For this reason, a candidate's publications form an important basis for assessing scholarly productivity.
>
> 1. *Research:* New knowledge can take many forms, including important clinical observations, clinical research findings, laboratory research, and integrative research.
>
> 2. *Teaching:* Excellence in teaching requires not only an objective, up-to-date, accurate, and balanced command of the field being taught but also effective communication skills. Course leadership and design, the judgment of students, trainees, and peers, and meritorious publications may also be considered when a faculty member's teaching is assessed.
>
> 3. *Clinical Distinction:* For faculty members who are clinicians, clinical distinction comprises professional excellence, integrity, and empathy in treating patients. Other elements of clinical distinction important for a faculty member's promotion include a national or international reputation, election to distinguished medical societies relevant to achievement in his or her field, the application of new knowledge, and meritorious publications.
>
> The following contributions will be considered by Promotion Committees in assessing faculty for advancement:

Teaching

—Quality and quantity of contact hours with students, including graduate students, medical students, residents, and postdoctoral fellows
—Educational program director for graduate students, medical students, residents, and postdoctoral fellows
—Development of new courses or special teaching materials, such as videotapes or computer material
—Teaching awards
—Directing or participating in continuing medical education courses

Publications

—Substantive and continuous publication in refereed journals with special emphasis on the quality of original contributions to the field
—Role of the faculty member in the execution of the project involved in the publications
—Number of authors and the place of the faculty member among the authors
—Textbooks or monographs—either as sole author or as editor
—Chapters in textbooks

Support for Research

—Grants and contracts obtained as the principal investigator or co-principal investigator
—Funding from grants and contracts with other principal investigators

National Recognition

—Awards or prizes for research or service
—Presentations at scholarly meetings and conferences
—Serving on national scientific advisory boards or study sections
—Serving as an officer or on the council of national scholarly organizations
—Membership in scholarly organizations
—Serving on editorial boards
—Invited presentations at universities, hospitals, etc.
—Organizing national and regional research meetings

Citizenship to the University

—Service on various university, School of Medicine, or department committees
—Serving as a division, program, or section chief

Clinical Service

—Reputation as a clinician, as manifested by referrals and peer review

—Number of clinic sessions and patients served
—Scope and productivity of clinical practice as compared to peers per-
forming similar services to similar patient populations
—Development of a unique or essential clinical program

Some faculty continue to be promoted primarily for their teaching activities since the adoption of the new policies.

The Grading System

One issue that was discussed a number of times during the planning and implementation stages of the new curriculum was our grading system. It was surprising to see how much strong emotion could be expressed over a topic related to adult learning and teaching. Johns Hopkins had always used letter grades (A to F) for all but a few courses that were graded as pass/fail. Many of the students and faculty members favored an honors/pass/fail system. This topic was debated in several EPC meetings during the year in which the new curriculum was being planned. By the time the new curriculum for the first year was implemented, the resolution was not to change the system but to decrease the number of grades per year because of the combining of courses. In addition, most courses were to add short, weekly quizzes to determine early in the process whether a student needed extra tutoring and to relieve the stress caused by determining grades on the basis of a few large examinations.

The first-year faculty felt very strongly that these alterations and the institution of small-group sessions would relieve the students' concern about grades. They and others who favored maintaining letter grades felt that the EPC's system allowed for better evaluation of students. This meant that a student's transcript and dean's letter would allow residency directors to better evaluate him or her. Our students' excellent record in matching for residencies, especially compared with the record of students at some sister schools that used a pass/fail system, was thought to be further proof that letter grades were best.

The topic of grades was revisited once, two years after the curriculum was implemented, but with nowhere near the emotion of the earlier discussions. We have maintained the letter grades, and no one has raised the topic, other than in passing, since that time. I am confident that this peace will not last forever.

Financial Issues

Since the implementation of our new curriculum would involve additional faculty time, we needed to address the issue of additional costs. When I accepted responsibility for overseeing the development and implementation of the new curriculum, the dean agreed that he would provide funding for the additional costs. While it would be very nice to have a grant, the grant monies would be available for only a limited time, and even during that time the funding would not cover all costs. Further, we would use the grant funds primarily for planning, pilots, and start-up costs.

Traditionally, the dean provided each department with general funds generated from a percentage of professional clinical fees. Some of these general fund monies were to be used to cover the cost of educating medical students. The problem was that there were no formulas or guidelines for how the monies were to be distributed. Therefore, every department director was free to make that determination with essentially no oversight from the dean's office. A quick study was performed to try to determine the relationships between the salary paid to faculty from general funds and the amount of time they spent teaching medical students. For the most part, there was no correlation. I am fairly certain that we are not alone among medical schools in having this disparity.

We have had several discussions in the dean's office regarding the feasibility of decreasing each department's general funds by a certain percentage and using those monies to directly reimburse those faculty whom we knew to be heavily involved in teaching medical students. We soon abandoned that idea when we considered the potential repercussions and the bad will that probably would result. We have also discussed the possibility of simply not increasing the general funds allocated each year and allocating the monies that would be saved by this decision to faculty who teach medical students. That plan also proved to be unfeasible because cutbacks meant that only the basic science departments would receive annual increases in general funds during the period when we were planning and implementing the curriculum. To the present we have made no change in the general funds allocation, but we agree that it makes good sense to centralize the remuneration of faculty for teaching medical students.

To determine reasonable additional costs, and therefore the allocation of grant monies and funding from the dean, I met individually with each of the directors or coordinators of the various components of the curriculum. The general guideline used was that there would be no additional financial remuneration for replacement courses or programs as long as essentially the same faculty time was involved. For example, a lump sum was set aside to help defray the costs of the small-group sessions in the first-year basic science courses. I asked Dr. Pollard to develop a formula that he and his group felt would be fair to reimburse each of the departments on the basis of the increased time needed to teach small groups. This allowed them to determine what they believed to be a fair allocation. This mechanism took pressure off the dean's office and eliminated one area in which the directors or faculty might have questioned the allocation of funds.

Additional funds were provided for the administrative time expended by new coordinators, secretarial support for each of the coordinators of the curriculum's first two years, and the directors of the two new courses—Physician and Society, and Introduction to Clinical Medicine. The program that required the bulk of the new funds was the Physician and Society course, which was a brand new course that spanned all four years of the curriculum and involved more than one hundred faculty. The money was used to reimburse faculty serving as module leaders and small-group leaders. We did not pay for the teaching of single class sessions because these involved so little time from any individual faculty member.

Relatively small amounts of money were allocated to remunerate the directors of the new courses, including the Introduction to Clinical Medicine, the Microbiology course, and the General Internal Medicine Ambulatory Rotation. One-time costs were covered for equipment to start the new Developmental Biology course in the first year. The other major costs included the start-up and ongoing costs of the Office of Medical Education Services and the Office of Medical Informatics Education.

During the years in which the new curriculum was being implemented, several gifts, grants, and contracts were obtained to augment the funding needed to attain our goals. Once the Clinical Education Center was fully operational, Dr. Shatzer was able to negotiate a number of contracts primarily for testing, using standardized patients. The contractors included several clinical departments (which paid for resident and postdoctoral fellow education), the Johns Hopkins University School of Nursing, the National Board of Medical Examiners, the Educational Commission on Foreign Medical Graduates, and a number of other medical schools and teaching hospitals. The profits from these contracts are used to defray the costs of educating our own students. Of course, any contract with the medical school departments was budget-neutral. That is, initiatives for resident and fellow education had to pay for themselves, but we made no profit on these projects. Dr. Lehmann was also successful in obtaining grants from the provost's office and from the National Library of Medicine for some projects of the Office of Medical Informatics Education.

Once the curriculum was ongoing and all grant funding ceased, the total increased cost to the dean's office was about $700,000 annually.

Changes in Leadership

Over the years, any program will experience changes in leadership, and ours was no exception. Ironically, most of the major changes occurred in 1996, after the index class graduated. Dean Johns and Dr. Pollard (the year 1 coordinator) accepted positions in other institutions, and Dr. Kidd (the year 2 coordinator) retired. Fortunately, we were able to fill the coordinator positions with faculty leaders who had been intimately involved in the respective programs. The leadership of the Introduction to Clinical Medicine course changed in 1995, and there were several changes in the coordinators of year 1 and years 3–4 of the Physician and Society course in 1994 and 1996; however, Dr. Gordis remained the overall director of Physician and Society. In all cases, the transitions were smooth, and each new leader brought fresh ideas and renewed vigor to the process.

These seamless transitions were viewed as evidence of a sound, institutionally based and supported effort that was not dependent on any single individual or individuals for success. The importance of this final point should not be underestimated. Any successful curriculum should be able to thrive no matter who the principals are.

Note

1. C. R. Taylor, "Occasional notes, great expectations: The reading habits of year II medical students," *New England Journal of Medicine* 326 (1992): 436–40.

3

Basic Sciences

THE FIRST YEAR
Thomas D. Pollard, M.D.

A group of basic scientists known as the First Year Basic Science Committee, or the first-year committee, formulated the basic science component of the new first-year curriculum during the winter and spring of 1992, and their decisions were implemented in September 1992. The charge to the committee was to evaluate the existing basic science curriculum and to recommend and implement revisions to strengthen the education of medical students. In consultation with the directors of the basic science departments and the leaders of the existing basic science courses, I selected a group of basic scientists with a commitment to education and expertise regarding the curriculum. The membership included every course director in the existing curriculum and represented all of the basic science departments (table 3.1). Except for me, none of the committee members was a departmental director. Dr. Catherine De Angelis, vice dean for academic affairs and faculty, or her designee, attended most meetings to keep the administration informed.

A retreat held early in 1992 was the pivotal event in the formulation of the basic science component of the new curriculum. This retreat allowed committee members to share experiences and to evaluate the existing curriculum. Although everyone was familiar with the existing schedule of courses (table 3.2), few had any detailed knowledge of the content and teaching methods of courses other than their own. In fact, some of the course directors had never met each other. The retreat allowed committee members to understand the full scope of the curriculum in greater detail than anyone had in the past. The subsequent effectiveness of the committee was due largely to the retreat, at which the group bonded together with a common purpose, empowered by our knowledge of the task at hand.

We retreated to a comfortable off-campus site on a Saturday to learn, in detail, what the medical students experienced during each day of their first year in

Table 3.1 Planning Committee for Basic Science in the New Curriculum

Professor	Department	Course Directed
S. Desiderio	Molecular Biology and Genetics	Microbiology
R. Dintzis	Cell Biology and Anatomy	Organ Histology
D. Fearon	Medicine	Immunology
B. Guggino	Physiology	Physiology
J. Hart	Biological Chemistry	Biochemistry
P. Murphy	Cell Biology and Anatomy	Organ Histology
T. Pollard	Cell Biology and Anatomy	Cells and Tissues
P. Rabins	Psychiatry and Behavioral Sciences	Behavioral Science
K. Rose	Cell Biology and Anatomy	Anatomy and Embryology
L. Schramm	Biomedical Engineering	Neuroscience
M. Steinmetz	Neuroscience	Neuroscience
P. Watkins	Neurology	Biochemical Nutrition

medical school. At about 8 A.M., we started with the first day of school in September and proceeded one day at a time through the whole year, until late that afternoon we reached the last examination in May. The course directors described briefly the content of each lecture, discussion group, laboratory, clinic, and examination. With the entire year of basic sciences on the table at one time, each participant could assess the strengths and weaknesses.

As we proceeded, committee members asked questions, challenged the relevance of some of the material, and commented on balance and scheduling. For example, our immunologist, whose clinical expertise is in rheumatology, argued that the Anatomy course placed far too much emphasis on the extremities and joints! Members also questioned whether all of the courses were appropriate for the first year. In particular, the director of the Behavioral Science course wondered whether his course might more appropriately be placed in the second year.

The chair of the second-year committee attended the retreat briefly. In retrospect, we should have included the entire second-year committee and urged them strongly to stay for the whole retreat, since the information exchange would have provided them with a novel perspective on the first year that would have been valuable to their efforts to improve the second year. A reciprocal event for us on the content of the second year would also have been valuable.

Our one-day survey of the content of the first-year basic science courses was reassuring but surprising, because our preconceived concerns about the curriculum turned out to be largely misplaced. Our weaknesses were largely unsuspected before we had the broad picture as well as detailed knowledge of the content of the first year.

This is what we found with respect to content:

1. There was remarkably little redundancy. This was unexpected, because no organized effort had ever been made to partition the content among the existing departmental courses. Apparently, individual faculty members had eliminated most duplication through ad hoc arrangements with colleagues in other departments. Feedback from students over the years also had contributed.

2. The coverage of basic science was relatively complete, but several deficiencies stood out. By contemporary standards we were short on genetics and molecular biology. We covered traditional embryology but offered nothing on the genetic, molecular, or cellular aspects of development.

3. Most courses made extensive use of disease processes to illustrate basic biology, but the students had little or no contact with either patients or practicing physicians.

4. Some topics were highly dispersed across the year rather than concentrated together where the general principles could be appreciated. For example, membrane physiology appeared in bits and pieces in cell biology (in the first quarter), neuroscience (in the third quarter), and organ physiology (in the fourth quarter).

This is what we learned about our approach to teaching and learning:

1. Each course used some excellent teaching, learning, and evaluation methods, but none of these methods was used across the board by the various courses. For example, Biochemistry scheduled discussions of classic research papers; Neuroscience wrapped up each week with a clinic to link the basic science with a relevant clinical problem; Cell Biology used low-stress weekly quizzes to help students keep up and to identify students with problems; and Microbiology used small groups to review lecture material and included student participation in the discussion as part of the evaluation of students.

2. Overall, 50 percent of the class time was scheduled for laboratories and small-group discussions, and 40 percent of the time was scheduled for lectures. The balance of the time was used for review and examination. Although the overall emphasis on lectures did not seem particularly excessive, as many as four lectures were scheduled on some days.

3. Except in examinations, students were rarely asked to solve problems.

4. The total amount of time spent in class (thirty-two hours per week) was excessive. Even worse, the time was not scheduled effectively; classes ran from 9 A.M. to noon and from 1 to 5 P.M. four days a week and from 9 A.M. to 1 P.M. the fifth day. Simply attending class was a full-time job for our students.

Table 3.2 Old First-Year Schedule

Time	Monday	Tuesday	Wednesday	Thursday	Friday
First Quarter (weeks 1–4), 9/5/91–10/4/91					
9 A.M.–12 noon	Biochemistry	Biochemistry	Biochemistry	Biochemistry	Biochemistry
12 noon–1 P.M.	Free	Free	Cells and Tissues[a]	Free	Free
1–5 P.M.	Cells and Tissues	Cells and Tissues	Free	Cells and Tissues	Cells and Tissues
First Quarter (weeks 5–9), 10/7/91–11/1/91					
9 A.M.–12 noon	Biochemistry	Biochemistry	Biochemistry	Biochemistry	Biochemistry
12 noon–1 P.M.	Free	Free	Anatomy and Embryology	Free	Free
1–5 P.M.	Anatomy and Embryology	Anatomy and Embryology	Free	Anatomy and Embryology	Anatomy and Embryology
Second Quarter (9 weeks), 11/4/91–1/10/92					
9–10 A.M.	Immunology/Microbiology[b]	Immunology/Microbiology	Immunology/Microbiology	Immunology/Microbiology	Immunology/Microbiology
10 A.M.–12 noon	Ethics and Medical Care	Immunology/Microbiology	Immunology/Microbiology	Immunology/Microbiology	Immunology/Microbiology
12 noon–1 P.M.	Free	Free	Immunology/Microbiology	Immunology/Microbiology	Free

(continued)

Table 3.2 (continued)

1–2 P.M.	Anatomy and Embryology	Anatomy and Embryology	Free	Free	Anatomy and Embryology
2–5 P.M.	Anatomy and Embryology	Anatomy and Embryology	Free	Ethics and Medical Care	Anatomy and Embryology
Third Quarter (9 weeks), 1/13/92–3/13/92					
9 A.M.–1 P.M.	Neuroscience	Neuroscience	Neuroscience	Neuroscience	Behavioral Science
2–5 P.M.	Behavioral Science	Behavioral Science	Free	Behavioral Science	Neuroscience
Fourth Quarter (9 weeks), 3/23/92–5/20/92					
9–10 A.M.	Physiology	Physiology	Physiology	Physiology	Physiology
10–11 A.M.	Physiology	Physiology/Organ Histology[c]	Biochemical Nutrition	Physiology	Biochemical Nutrition
11 A.M.–1 P.M.	Physiology	Physiology/Organ Histology	Physiology	Physiology	Physiology
2–5 P.M.	Physiology	Emergency Medicine[d]	Organ Histology	Physiology	Physiology

[a]Cells and Tissues: Wednesday lecture met from 12:30 to 1:30 P.M.

[b]Immunology/Microbiology: These two courses met for three weeks and six weeks, respectively.

[c]Physiology/Organ Histology: These two courses met in four sessions each; sequence was determined by course director.

[d]Emergency Medicine met for eight required sessions; additional elective sessions were offered.

5. Given the demands of the schedule, students rarely found the time to read books and, with few exceptions, read little or no original literature. Their learning generally was confined to what they heard in class or read in the lecture notes provided by each of the courses.

6. Scheduling of examinations was counterproductive. Not only did some examinations compete with each other for the students' attention, but examinations invariably diverted the attention of the students from concurrent courses.

We used several other sources to refine and reinforce these conclusions about the strengths and weaknesses of the first year. Most departments had solicited student critiques of their courses over the previous decade and had modified their courses to some extent to deal with specific student concerns. This new revision of the curriculum as a whole allowed them to deal with large-scale systemic problems such as the conflict between examinations and class activities and the congestion of the whole first year.

Committee members met regularly with a volunteer Student Curriculum Committee of seventeen first-year students during 1991/92. At these meetings, faculty members learned for the first time about student criticisms of courses other than their own. The students provided course evaluations and critiques of each quarter as the year progressed. While no student formally served on the first-year committee, we consulted the student committee frequently for advice as our ideas developed and our plans unfolded. The Student Curriculum Committee enthusiastically endorsed the plans for the new first year. Independently, the vice dean for academic affairs organized third- and fourth-year students to compile recommendations for our committee. Remarkably, their ideas were nearly identical to those of the faculty and the first-year students.

Members of the first-year committee reported frequently to their departments, and I also briefed the basic science directors independently, so that the faculty was kept informed about the findings of the committee and could provide additional suggestions about the impending changes in the curriculum. Two members of the first-year committee served on the committee that organized the new Physician and Society course (see chapter 5). This provided communication between the committees, but the two groups did not succeed in coordinating their activities to any meaningful extent. For example, it would have been desirable to schedule Physician and Society activities relevant to the ongoing content of the basic science courses, but the schedules of the courses were generally incompatible.

Several earlier experiments in individual courses also influenced the committee. For example, the Brieger committee (authors of the Brieger Report, discussed in chapter 1) had recommended a regular "journal club" in which the medical students would read original research papers. About one third of the first-year class in 1989/90 had volunteered for an experimental journal club. Both the students and the participating faculty were strongly positive about the club's value. Also, in an effort to discourage memorization and to encourage reading and thinking, open-book examinations had been used experimentally in the Cell Biology course. The reaction was generally positive, although some students expressed concern because they were not sure how to prepare for an examination in which no importance was placed on memorization.

Planning the New Basic Science Curriculum

Remarkably, the retreat crystallized the thinking of the first-year committee so effectively that by the time the retreat ended we were all committed to a common vision for the curriculum. This consensus occurred with little debate, because once we all saw the big picture as well as our strengths and weaknesses, it was relatively obvious what we should do. In subsequent meetings we outlined our goals for the basic science courses (table 3.3) and the guiding principles (table 3.4) that would enable us to achieve these goals. This prepared us to begin planning for implementation.

The committee aimed to give students a high standard of proficiency in basic science, a goal rooted in the conviction that malfunctions in virtually every cellular process will eventually be recognized as contributing to human disease. We wanted to provide a high level of content delivered in a stimulating format. By making problem solving a high priority, we hoped to help students not only to understand the general principles of basic biomedical science but also to ac-

Table 3.3   Goals for the Basic Science Courses

The basic science courses should enable students to
   1. establish a long-term interest in basic biomedical science;
   2. develop skill and confidence in reading the original literature in contemporary biology;
   3. understand the general principles currently used to explain how humans function, form the molecular and cellular levels to the integration of organ systems;
   4. recognize the limits of contemporary knowledge of biology; and
   5. appreciate the potential of continued research at the cellular and molecular levels to contribute to the diagnosis, treatment, and prevention of disease.

Table 3.4   Guiding Principles of New First-Year Curriculum

---

1. Give students more responsibility for learning the assigned material outside class.
2. Encourage active learning.
3. Decompress the schedule.
4. Redesign content in a contemporary context rather than in a historical disciplinary content.
5. Put all of the content on the table for reorganization into new courses.
6. Start with molecules and finish with organ systems.
7. Strenghthen genetics, molecular biology, developmental biology, and cell physiology.
8. Move medical microbiology, emergency medicine, and nutrition to year 2.
9. Assign responsibility for the new, integrated courses to individual departments, but encourage participation by members of more than one department in each course.
10. Reduce stress in student evaluations.
11. Consolidate exams to avoid conflicts with teaching schedule.
12. Use open-book exams where feasible.
13. Implement the new curriculum in September 1992, whether or not the final details are settled.

---

quire the skills required to solve problems or propose hypotheses when no concrete answer is known.

Guided by these goals and general principles, it was relatively easy to piece together the new curriculum. We conceptualized the educational process in three separate parts: (1) an overall plan for logical coverage of the content; (2) detailed assignment of material to different courses; and (3) daily and weekly schedules of stimulating activities to facilitate our educational goals.

The Logic behind the New Basic Science Curriculum

We quickly agreed to start with macromolecules, and then move on to cells and finally to organ systems (table 3.5). Anatomy and Developmental Biology were inserted after Molecules and Cells and before Organ Systems, because Developmental Biology depends upon the concepts of cellular and molecular biology and understanding of organ systems depends upon knowledge of gross anatomy. During the first two years in which the new curriculum was implemented, Developmental Biology overlapped with Anatomy, but after that we settled on separate blocks, with Anatomy followed by a two-week block of Developmental Biology. Immunology was hard to place, but it finally ended up as one of the organ systems. We have never resolved whether it is better to cover the nervous system

Table 3.5   Block Outline of the First Year

Block	Weeks	Dates
I. Molecules and Cells[a]	12	Labor Day to Thanksgiving
II. Anatomy; Developmental Biology[b]	11	Thanksgiving to end of January
III. Neuroscience; Epidemiology[c]	8	Mid-February to mid-April
IV. Organ Systems[d]	10	First two weeks of February; mid-April to mid-June

[a]Block I. Molecules and Cells. This large course is divided into four sections: two weeks of Macromolecules (responsibility of the Department of Biophysics and Biophysical Chemistry), three weeks of Molecular Biology and Genetics (responsibility of the Department of Molecular Biology and Genetics), three weeks of Cell Physiology (joint responsibility of the Department of Cell Biology and Anatomy and the Department of Physiology), and three weeks part time of Metabolism (responsibility of the Department of Biological Chemistry).

[b]Block II. Anatomy; Developmental Biology. The Anatomy course is the responsibility of the Department of Cell Biology and Anatomy. It is followed by a two-week course in Developmental Biology taught by an interdepartmental committee.

[c]Block III. Neuroscience; Epidemiology. The Neuroscience course is the responsibility of the Department of Neuroscience. A concurrent course in Epidemiolgy is the responsibility of the Department of Epidemiology of the school of hygiene and public health.

[d]Block IV. Organ Systems. This course consists of two weeks of Immunology (responsibility of the Department of Medicine) scheduled for the first two weeks of February, before block III; and eight weeks of integrated coverage of the cardiovascular, pulmonary, renal, gastrointestinal, endocrine, and reproductive systems (responsibility of the departments of Physiology, Biomedical Engineering, and Cell Biology and Anatomy), scheduled to follow block III from mid-April to mid-June.

before or after the other organ systems. We have tried it both ways; each has advantages, but none are overriding.

To concentrate faculty effort and to avoid competition between courses and examinations, we generally have used block courses. Some faculty were initially concerned about the scheduling of their course as a short, stand-alone block, fearing that too little time would be available for students to assimilate the material. However, this generally has not been a problem, and there are clear advantages for students in focusing their full attention on one subject at a time. One exception to block scheduling is that the Anatomy course begins during the last three weeks of Molecules and Cells. This allows students to ease into this most unfamiliar part of their studies and spreads out the study of metabolism enough to keep it from being too burdensome for either the students or the faculty. A second exception is the scheduling of Epidemiology during the Neuroscience course. Spreading out Neuroscience has practical advantages in terms of scheduling laboratories and miniprojects with individual faculty members.

The Creation of New Courses with Redefined Departmental Responsibilities

Next we assigned the curriculum content to the various blocks. Since the content of the whole year was all "on the table" for the first time, the first-year committee found it relatively easy to fit each topic into a logical progression. Although this resulted in significant changes from the existing departmental courses, and reassignments of responsibility, it was accomplished without significant concerns about departmental territory. This was possible because everyone on the committee was informed about the big picture and was more committed to presenting a coherent course of study than to preserving traditional departmental teaching assignments.

To create the new curriculum, we rearranged pieces of the old curriculum. For example, to put together an integrated unit on membrane physiology, we moved material on pumps, carriers, channels, and membrane excitability from the old Neuroscience course and the Renal unit of the old Physiology course to the new Cell Physiology block of the Molecules and Cells course, where it was integrated with material on membrane biogenesis and membrane traffic (all from the old Cells and Tissues course). Material on the development of blood cells and bones was moved from the old Cells and Tissues course to the new Developmental Biology course. For the first time, we provided extensive coverage of macromolecular structure and many aspects of genetics during the first two blocks of the new Molecules and Cells course. The old Physiology and Histology courses were combined into one Organ Systems course, under the leadership of the Department of Physiology, but with heavy participation of cell biologists for the teaching of microscopic anatomy. The content of some parts of the curriculum did not change. The old Neuroscience course was already a model of integrated content, so most of it remained intact.

The new sequence of subject matter is certainly more logical than the old one, but four years of experience have revealed that we can do better. For example, the presentation of cellular signal transduction mechanisms is still fragmented and incomplete. We continue to work on it.

Everyone agreed that departmental ownership of and responsibility for teaching activities is essential for faculty commitment to high-quality teaching, so responsibility for each section of the new curriculum is assigned to a specific department (table 3.5). The only exception is the new Developmental Biology course, which is run by a committee of faculty from several departments. We encourage departments, when arranging the curricular segments for which they are responsible, to recruit appropriate faculty from other departments to help with the teaching. One example is the first two weeks of Molecules and Cells. The Department of Biophysics and Biophysical Chemistry is in charge of the section on macromolecules, but the teaching faculty also come from the Department of Biological Chemistry and the Department of Cell Biology and Anatomy. All of the involved departments recognize participation in the section on macromolecules as a valuable contribution of their faculty toward fulfilling their responsibility to medical student teaching.

With the block schedule, most faculty are committed to one or two sections of teaching, each of which lasts two to three weeks. The anatomists have a ten-week commitment (three weeks part-time, seven full-time). For the duration of each of these blocks, faculty members are committed essentially to full-time teaching, since class activities extend from 8 A.M. to 1 P.M. Ideally (and in practice for most courses), participating faculty members attend all of the lectures. Between the lectures, each faculty member is responsible for a small group in discussion or laboratory sessions. During the afternoons, additional time is usually required for the faculty and teaching assistants to prepare the discussion groups or laboratories for the next day. Compared with the old curriculum, this represents a larger teaching commitment and much more personal responsibility for the material in a course. For some faculty, a lack of familiarity with the details of all aspects of their subject created anxiety the first time through the discussion groups, but they gained confidence with experience.

The Weekly Schedule: Success Is in the Details

Our most important decisions dealt with the practical details embodied in the revised weekly schedule (table 3.6). How could we simultaneously encourage more active learning, decompress the schedule, reduce stress about examinations, and introduce original research literature? We made some general decisions about the smallest details first and then worried about the schedule for the year as a whole. We were enthusiastic about an administrative decision to include two new courses that provided first-year students with their first experiences with medical practice: two hours per week for the new Physician and Society course and one afternoon every other week for Introduction to Clinical Medicine, the new preceptorship with practicing physicians.

First, we decided to eliminate afternoon basic science classes to free up a large block of time on most days for individual study. We tried to fit all of our activities between 9 A.M. and 1 P.M., but this proved to be impossible. This drove us to a crucial decision—to start the day at 8 A.M. It seemed radical at the time, but this key decision has served us well, making unscheduled afternoons a reality without any undue inconvenience to students or faculty. The unscheduled afternoons are essential to provide adequate time to students for reading,

Table 3.6   Revised Weekly Schedule

Time	Monday	Tuesday	Wednesday	Thursday	Friday
8:00 A.M.	Lecture	Lecture	Lecture	Lecture	Lecture
9:30 A.M.	Discussion/ lab[a]	Journal club[b]	Discussion/ lab	Discussion/ lab	Discussion/ lab
10:30 A.M.		Discussion/			
11:00 A.M.		lab	PAS[c]		
11:45 A.M.	Lecture	Lecture	PAS	Lecture	Lecture
1:00 P.M.	Free	Free	Free	Free	Free
2:00 P.M.					Clinical Correlations[d]

[a]Discussion/lab: small-group discussion of problem sets, or lab taught to group of fifteen students.

[b]Journal club: a weekly meeting of fifteen students at which a paper is read from the current literature relevant to the students' current courses. The students discuss the paper with a junior faculty member from a clinical department and rotating faculty from the basic science departments (two faculty per session).

[c]PAS: Physician and Society course.

[d]Clinical Correlations: a Friday clinic involving a patient presentation, an analysis of clinical features, and a strong basic science component designed to integrate the main concepts covered during the week.

preparing problem sets, taking advantage of computerized learning facilities, discussing work with classmates, visiting physicians' offices as part of Introduction to Clinical Medicine, and participating in some volunteer activities.

Second, we decided to schedule only two lectures per day, generally at the beginning (8:00 A.M.) and end (11:45 A.M.) of class time. This has worked well. We are flexible on the timing (so that the anatomy laboratory can run to the end of class time at 1:00 P.M.) but have no exceptions to our rule of only two lectures per day. These lectures are supported by detailed lecture notes in outline form, which provide most of the factual material on each topic. Most of the lecture notes are illustrated; some, but not all, of the diagrams and micrographs are projected as slides or overheads during the lecture. Thus, students need not take detailed notes during lecture and instead can concentrate on understanding the arguments and examples used by the lecturer to illustrate the main points. Most students preview the lecture notes before the lectures. This is important because the lectures generally are fast paced and are presented on a high level.

Third, between the two lectures, we scheduled time for small-group discussions and laboratories. These are quite varied, but include discussions of problem sets in most courses (see table 3.7 for examples of discussion questions); microscopy laboratories in the Cell Physiology, Neuroscience, and Organ Systems

Table 3.7 Sample Small-Group Discussion Questions from the Molecules and Cells Course

1. If you were to redesign life but were allowed to use only 15 amino acids, which ones would you choose, and why? What if you could use only 10? Are there side-chains that are not used that you would add to the repertoire? Why are there as many/few as 20, anyway? (There are no right answers to these questions, but they are interesting to think about.)

2. Assume that a given protein binds to DNA and bends the DNA toward the protein. How would the equilibrium binding constant change if the DNA were pre-bent in this manner? How would the binding constnat change if the DNA were pre-bent in the opposite direction?

3. Familial retinoblastoma is said to be an autosomal dominant condition, yet it arises only when *both* alleles are defective or deleted. How do you explain this apparent discrepancy?

4. The presence in the same cell of a normal p53 allele and an allele with a specific point mutation in the p53 gene can lead to cell transformation to tumorigenicity. How can you explain this "dominant negative" effect of the mutation?

5. You want to express high levels of a protein from a gene you have cloned so that you can study the protein biochemically. The gene codes for a cytoplasmic enzyme. You decide to express the protein in yeast, and you construct a vector that places the coding sequence in your cDNA behind a cleavable signal sequence so that the protein will be secreted and you can purify it from the medium. Using this vector, you find that yeast cells synthesize large amounts of your protiein and that it is translocated into the yeast ER (endoplasmic reticulum). However, it fails to leave the ER, and there is no enzymatic activity when cell homogenates are assayed. What are some possible explanations?

6. Nearly 100 different myosin heavy chain point mutations have been detected as genetic causes of hypertrophic cardiomyopathy. All of the mutations are located in the head or subfragment-2 domains, none in the light meromysin. Since mutations should occur randomly, how can you account for the distribution of the mutations?

Note: Many students prepare written answers to the questions; some discuss the questions with classmates before class.

courses; and gross anatomy dissections and wet laboratories in the Molecular Biology and Genetics, Immunology, and Organ Systems courses. See table 3.8 for examples of wet laboratories. For the first semester, we divided the students into small groups of fifteen according to their self-assessed backgrounds in science (advanced, intermediate, and elementary). They were randomly assigned to new groups for the second semester.

Fourth, we added a journal club on Tuesdays after the lecture for each discussion group of fifteen students. The students read a short, contemporary re-

Table 3.8   Examples of Wet Laboratory Topics

Molecular Biology and Genetics
    Pneumococcal transformatnion
    Superinfection immunity
    Detection of sickle cell mutations
    Loss of heterozygosity
Immunology
    Antibody formation
    Polymerase chain reaction
    Mechanisms of thymic selection
    Lymphoid tissues
Organ Systems
    Renal-electrolyte physiology
    Respiratory physiology
    Cardiovasuclar physiology

---

search paper related to the scientific content of the previous week. See table 3.9 for a list of papers that were discussed in each of the journal clubs in 1995/96. Each journal club meets for about fifty minutes with two faculty members to discuss the methods, results, and interpretation of the paper that is under discussion that week. One of these faculty members is from a clinical department and stays with the group for the whole semester. The other is the basic scientist who leads the discussion group for that block of the course. The object is to acquire the technical knowledge and critical skills required to read the research literature.

Fifth, we added a Clinical Correlations class each Friday afternoon. This is the only violation of our rule against afternoon classes. These clinics cover a topic related to the basic science material covered each week. See table 3.10 for a listing of topics covered in Clinical Correlations. A clinical faculty member presents a patient and gives a short talk on the clinical manifestations and molecular basis of the patient's disease. Students question the patient or the patient's family about the disease and how it has affected their lives. The clinics illustrate the immediate relevance of basic science to health and disease and reinforce the importance of basic biology for physicians who aspire to advance medical knowledge.

The model weekly schedule, as shown in table 3.6, is followed with some variation throughout the year. This new curriculum week has twenty-three hours of basic science class, compared with thirty-two hours in the old curriculum. Given the two extra hours of Physician and Society and the two new hours of Clinical Correlations, the new schedule has only one less hour per day than the old, but the students' time is used much more effectively because most after-

Table 3.9   Journal Club Articles, 1995/96

Molecules and Cells

Week 1   Rouault, T. A., et al. "Structural relationship between an iron-regulated REN-binding protein (IRE-BP) and aconitase: Functional implications." *Cell* 64 (1991):881–83.

Week 2   Lam, P. Y. S., et al. "Rational design of potent, bioavailable, nonpeptide cyclic ureas as HIV protease inhibitors." *Science* 263 (1994): 380–84.

Week 3   Cho, Y., et al. "Crystal structure of a p53 tumor suppressor-DNA complex: Understanding tumorigenic mutations." *Science* 165 (1994): 346–55.

Week 4   Smith, H. O., et al. "Frequency and distribution of DNA uptake signals in the H. influenzae in the Rd genome." *Science* 269 (1995):538–39.

Background reading to prepare for week 5: Fleishman, R. D., et al. "Whole genome random sequencing and assembly of Haemophilus influenzae Rd." *Science* 269 (1995):496–512.

Week 5   Savitsky, K., et al. "A single ataxia telangiectasia gene with a product similar to PI-3 kinase." *Science* 268 (1995):1749–53.

Week 6   Laird, P., et al. "Suppression of intestinal neoplasia by DNA hypomethylation." *Cell* 81 (1995):197–205.

Week 7   Sparkowski, J., J. Anders, and R. Schlege. "E5 oncoprotein retained in the endoplasmic reticulum/cis Golgi still induces PDGF receptor autophosphorylation but does not transform cells." *EMBO Journal* 14 (1995):3055–63.

Week 8   Nakai, J., et al. "Restoration of both excitation-contraction coupling and slow Ca^{2+} current in dispedic muscle by skeletal ryanodine receptor cDNA." *Nature* 336 (1988):134–39.

Week 9   Theriot, J., et al. "The rate of actin-based motility of intracellualr Listeria monocytogenes equals the rate of actin polymerization." *Nature* 357 (1992):257–60.

Week 10   Epstein, P., et al. "Expression of yeast hexokinase in pancreatic B cells of transgenic mice reduces blood glucose, enhances insulin secretion, and decreases diabetes." *Proceedings of the National Academy of Sceinces USA* 89 (1992):12038–42.

Week 11   Halaas, J., et al. "Weight-reducing effects of the plasma protein encoded by the obese gene." *Science* 269 (1994):543–47.

Developmental Biology

January 16   Handyside, A., et al. "Birth of a normal girl after fertilization and preimplantation diagnostic testing for cystic fibrosis." *New England Journal of Medicine* 327 (1992):905–9.

(continued)

Table 3.9   *(continued)*

January 23	Levin, M., et al. "A molecular pathway determining left-right asymmetry in chick embryogenesis." *Cell* 82 (1995):803–14.
Immunology	
January 30	Kuo, Choo, et al. "Isolation of a cDNA clone derived from a bloodborne non-A, non-B viral hepatitis genome." *Science* 244 (1989): 359–62.
	Kuo, Choo, et al. "An assy for circulating antibodies to a major etiologic virus of human non-A, non-B hepatitis." *Science* 244 (1989): 362–64.
February 6	Bordignon, C., et al. "Gene therapy in peripheral blood lymphocytes and bone marrow for ADA-immunodeficient patients." *Science* 270 (1995):356–61.
Neuroscience	
February 13	Levi-Mantalcini, R., and B. Booker. "Destruction of the sympathetic ganglia in mammals by antiserum to a nerve growth protein." *Proceedings of the National Academy of Sciences USA* 46 (1960):384–91.
February 20	Toyka, K.V., et al. "Myasthenia gravis: Passive transfer from man to mouse." *Science* 190 (1975): 397–99.
February 27	"Lesion of striatal neurons with kainic acid provides a model for Huntington's chorea." *Nature* 263 (1976):244–46.
March 5	Pons, T. P., et al. "Massive cortical reorganization after sensory deafferentiation in adult macaques." *Science* 252 (1991):1857–60.
March 12	Kinomura, S., et al. "Activation by attention of the human reticular formation and thalamic intralaminar nuclei." *Science* 271 (1996):512–15.
March 26	Langston J. W., et al. "Chronic Parkinson in humans due to a product of neperidine-analog synthesis." *Science* 219 (1983):979–80.
April 2	Buch, L., and R. Axel. "A novel multigene family may encode odorant receptors: A molecular basis for odor recognition." *Cell* 65 (1991): 175–87.
April 9	Tallal, P., et al. "Language comprehension in language-learning impaired children improved with acoustically modified speech." *Science* 271 (1996):81–84.
Organ systems	
April 16	Reichard, P., et al. "The effect of long-term intesified insulin treatment on the development of microvascular complications of diabetes mellitus." *New England Journal of Medicine* 329 (1993):304–9.

(continued)

Table 3.9   (*continued*)

April 30	Smith J. C., et al. "Pre-Botzinger complex: A brainstem region that may generate respiratory rhythm in mammals." *Science* 254 (1991): 726–29.
May 7	Schwartz, P., et al. "Long QT syndrome patients with mutations of the SCN5A and HERG genes have differential responses to Na$^+$ channel blockade and to increases in heart rate." *Circulation* 92 (1995): 3381–86.
	Rosen, M. R. "Long QT syndrome patients with gene mutations." *Circulation* 92 (1995):3373–75.
May 14	Chang, M., et al. "Adenovirus-mediated over-expression of the cyclin/cyclin-dependent kinase inhibitor, p21, inhibits vascular smooth muscle cell proliferation and neointima formation in the rat carotid artery model of balloon angioplasty." *Journal of Clinical Investigation* 96 (1995):2260–68.
May 21	Bhaskar, K. R. "Viscous fingering of HCL through gastric mucin." *Nature* 360 (1992):458–62.
	Walsbren, S. "Unusual permeability properties of gastric gland cells." *Nature* 368 (1994):332–35.
May 28	Marchetti, M. "Development of a mouse model of Helicobaster pylori infection that mimics human disease." *Science* 267 (1995):1655–58.
June 4	Matthews, C. H., et al. "Primary amenorrhea and infertility due to a mutation in the b-subunit of follicle-stimulating hormone." *Nature Genetics* 5 (1993):83–86.

noons (in addition to weekends and evenings) are free for studying or other activities.

During the reorganization, some old material was condensed or replaced, but a significant amount of new material was added to make up for our deficiencies in genetics and developmental biology, so some adjustments had to be made to fit the new schedule within the academic year. We started by moving Medical Microbiology and Nutrition to the second year. Later we moved Behavioral Science to the second year to compensate for including in Epidemiology some new material on biostatistics. Nevertheless, we had to extend the first year by about three weeks, until the middle of June. This caused some minor hardships, but it is generally felt that the decompression of the weekly schedule has made it worthwhile.

The first-year committee never wrote an extensive report on any of our ac-

Table 3.10 Topics Covered in Clinical correlations in 1995/96

Molecules and Cells
  Sickle cell anemia
  Xeroderma pigmentosa
  Disorders of DNA repair
  Cystic fibrosis
  Colon cancer
  Lysosomal diseases
  Muscular dystrophy
  Marfan syndrome
  Myasthenia gravis
  Glycogen storage disease
  Diabetes
  Abnormal serum lipids
Anatomy
  Facial deformities
  Extremities
  Thorax and chest
Developmental Biology
  Assisted reproduction technologies
  Neural tube defects
  Congenital heart disease
  Achondroplasias
  Genital malformations
  The fetus as a patient
Immunology
  Autoimmunity
  AIDS
Neuroscience
  AIDS neuropathy
  Poliolike illness
  Brain tumors
  Aneurysms
  Vertigo
  Psychotic disorders
  Motor diseases
Organ Systems
  Polycystic kidney disease
  Liver disease
  Asthma
  Respiratory distress syndrome
  Congenital complete heart block
  Shock
  Endocrines
  Male and female infertility

tivities or recommendations. The longest document that we produced prior to this chapter was a two-page summary of the general principles and the overall plan for the year. A summary was also used in the annual reports to the Robert Wood Johnson Foundation, which provided support for the curriculum revision. We found that personal briefings and consultations were an effective way to generate widespread support for reforms. The absence of a written report may have contributed to the lack of any organized opposition to our changes.

Implementation of the New Basic Science Curriculum

Although we started relatively late in the academic year, the first-year committee decided to implement the new curriculum in September 1992, even before all the details had been worked out. Although this created some anxiety, it was a wise decision because the high level of faculty interest and enthusiasm might have dissipated if we had delayed a full year. Furthermore, rapid implementation avoided any organized resistance to the changes that might have developed over time.

Although the first-year committee was firmly committed to the general principles and weekly format outlined above, we were quite flexible about some things. For example, the original plan called for Neuroscience and Behavioral Science to share the third quarter—despite some reservations, noted above, about the placement of Behavioral Science in the first year. Well into the first quarter, the second-year committee invited the Behavioral Science course to join the new second-year curriculum. To make time in the second year, the committee suggested that Epidemiology move to the first year. Due to faculty commitments, the only way to accommodate this change was to switch the third and fourth quarters of the first year. Thus, in December 1992, with less than eight weeks to go before the third quarter, we rescheduled the Organ Systems course for the third quarter and the combination of Neuroscience and Epidemiology for the fourth quarter. It is a tribute to the flexibility of our faculty that everything ran smoothly. At the request of the Department of Neuroscience, we reversed the order of the third and fourth quarters for the second iteration of the new curriculum, and Neuroscience and Epidemiology subsequently were placed between two segments of Organ Systems (table 3.5).

The implementation of the new basic science curriculum lay largely in the hands of the departments, particularly the faculty members assigned to direct the various courses. As the first-year basic science coordinator, I provided some overall guidance, resolved questions about educational philosophy and policy, chaired meetings of the course directors with the Student Curriculum Committee, and negotiated with the administration for support for innovations. All of this took less than 5 percent of my time. I was assisted ably by a half-time administrative assistant who coordinated the activities of the various courses, the journal club, and the clinics. This individual, who was partially funded by the dean's office, was absolutely essential to keep the first year running smoothly.

Evaluation of Students

Examinations were one of the greatest sources of student anxiety and of conflicts between courses in the old curriculum, and we sought ways to minimize both problems. Scheduling the courses one at a time in blocks immediately solved the problem of competition between examinations and class activities in concurrent courses. It also eliminated conflicts between closely scheduled examinations.

We retained the letter grades (A, B, C, D, F) that were traditional at Johns Hopkins, based on hour-long examinations at the end of each segment of a course and on performance in discussion groups. Timing of these examinations was based on subject matter. For example, each of the four parts of the Molecules and Cells course had an hour-long examination, the results of which were pooled to arrive at a grade for the course. Long courses such as Anatomy had several hour-long exams but no comprehensive final examination. In the Organ Systems course, material on physiology and histology was included in each of several hour-long examinations. Students received a grade for each quarter, i.e., for Molecules and Cells, for Anatomy and Developmental Biology, for Neuroscience, and for Organ Systems. Epidemiology was graded separately from Neuroscience, although it occupied a minor part of the same quarter. The committee recommended that student participation in small-group discussions be considered in grading, and in most courses this is now 25 to 33 percent of the final grade.

While the first-year committee issued no mandate, we asked each course to offer short, weekly, low-stress quizzes to keep students informed about their progress. During most weeks, students have a fifteen-minute quiz that counts little toward their grade. This enables faculty to identify any students struggling with the material and to provide help well before the student fails an important examination.

To reduce the anxiety surrounding examinations, the committee also asked the course directors to experiment with open-book examinations. The objective was to eliminate memorization and to test for integrative and creative thinking on examinations. In all courses except Anatomy, open-book examinations were tried during the first year, although Neuroscience eventually returned to a closed-book format on the premise that some memorization may be desirable. The

Table 3.11   Sample Examination Questions from the Molecules and Cells Course

1. The following three articles were published recently. Taking into account what you have learned, write a brief abstract (sixty words or fewer) describing the possible contents of one of these articles. Obviously, you do not know the actual content of the articles, so use your imagination.
   a. Gating Charge Differences between Two Voltage-Gated K^+ Channels Are Due to the Specific Charge Content of Their Respective S4 Regions
   b. Dictyostelium Myosin Heavy Chain Phosphorylation Sites Regulate Myosin Filament Assembly and Localization in Vivo
   c. Common Signals Control Low-Density Lipoprotein Receptor Sorting in Endosomes and the Golgi Complex of MDCK Cells
2. Suppose action potentials pass over a skeletal muscle fiber at intervals of 1 per sec. Will this have a significant effect on glucose transport by a uniport system (facilitated diffusion) or Ca^{2+} extrusion by $3Na^+/Ca^{2+}$: antiport (exchange)? If so, why? If not, why not?
   a. Glucose transport
   b. Ca^{2+} extrusion
3. The ER and Golgi complex disassemble into small vesicles (vesiculate) during mitosis, and secretion stops. Using your knowledge of vesicular transport and the cell cycle, briefly propose a mechanism that could account for the disassembly and subsequent assembly of mitotic organelles.
4. Osteogenesis imperfecta is an example of a human disease in which mutations in collagen produce a dominant negative phenotype. Name two proteins other than collagen where a mutation might produce a dominant negative phenotype. For each protein, explain (a) the molecular mechanism for the defect, and (b) the effect of this defect on the cell (or the human body).
5. If you were designing a microtubule-based motor protein that had to work alone or in cooperation with a small number of identical motor proteins associated with cargo (such as a small vesicle or an RNA particle), what kind of enzyme mechanism would you use? The point is to explain how a small number of motors can move a particle at a steady rate over long distances without falling off the microtubule.

   Use what you know about the actomyosin ATPase cycle, but modify the relative rates of the reaction to allow the motor to work more or less alone. Hint: Draw a diagram of the ATPase mechanism, using K for kinesin, M for microtubule, T for ATP, D for ADP, and P for phospohate. Then fill in arrows proportional to the approximate size of the rate constants for each forward and backward reaction. Indicate which intermediates are tightly bound to the microtubule and where free energy might be released to power the movement. Finally, explain why your mechanism is more appropriate for a vesicle motor than for muscle contraction.

committee also urged the faculty to minimize the length of examinations; previous examinations had been up to four hours long and it was clear that one could determine whether a student had mastered the material with a sixty- to ninety-minute examination. Keeping to a reasonably short time was essential for open-book examinations, in which the books were to be used as a reference for details, not to supply answers to questions on unfamiliar matierial. Compliance with this recommendation has been good but not uniform. We have maintained our tradition of problem solving or short essays for examinations, with essentially no true/false or multiple-choice questions. See table 3.11 for examples.

Evaluation of the New Basic Science Curriculum

Students and faculty have worked together since the implementation of the new curriculum to evaluate its strengths and weaknesses, with the goal of correcting any problems and reinforcing the successful elements. We have used the traditional written surveys and two kinds of new face-to-face meetings for these evaluations.

Written surveys. The developers of each section of the curriculum have solicited student opinions on written questionnaires. The course directors have shared the results with other members of the first-year committee, but the details regarding individual faculty evaluations have remained confidential. The students have also surveyed their classmates and the faculty; their findings are summarized in chapter 9.

Face-to-face meetings. Students select a representative from each discussion group for the Student Curriculum Committee. These representatives gather opinions from their classmates to provide the faculty with advise about each part of the new curriculum. Usually the students summarize their likes, dislikes, and suggestions in writing for each meeting with the faculty. A midcourse meeting with the course director and the first-year coordinator provides us with an interim assessment and allows for immediate adjustments if required. A similar meeting at the completion of each course provides an opportunity to plan for the next year. The meetings have been very constructive, with many suggestions for improvements in each course and little disagreement between students and faculty about what should be done. The course directors generally have been responsive and have implemented most of the student suggestions for the following year.

The course directors have continued to meet annually for assessment and large-scale planning. Student representatives attend one meeting to review the whole year. Other meetings are used to share experiences, to correct some organizational problems, and to optimize the sequence of material and the use of the time. We had hoped to cut at least one week off the year, but this has proved impossible thus far.

Broadly speaking, the faculty and students liked the following features of the new basic science curriculum:

1. The weekly format with afternoons free for reading, study, and outside activities.
2. Small-group discussions of problem sets. We have been impressed with how strongly the members of the groups bond together.
3. The journal club, provided that the paper is appropriate and an orientation sheet is available to introduce the topic.
4. The Friday afternoon Clinical Correlations class, provided that patients are included.
5. Detailed lecture notes with objectives, review questions, and figures embedded in the text.
6. Weekly quizzes.
7. Open-book examinations for appropriate courses. Courses with a heavy anatomical content (Anatomy and Neuroscience) use closed-book examinations.
8. Faculty commitment to and enthusiasm for the new format, including small-group discussions. Most faculty must work harder but find the experience to be more rewarding.
9. Computer learning where available. During the first two years, both computer hardware and software were limited, but their availability is expanding each year.
10. Integration of the material from formerly separate courses.

The students and/or faculty were concerned about the following problems:

1. Faculty anxiety and burnout in some blocks led to student anxiety. With experience, most faculty became confident about their teaching responsibilities, so this problem is now minimal.
2. Students were disappointed that some courses offered only limited problem sets and discussion groups. At their urging, most courses now include a substantial number of problem sets and discussions.
3. Some courses did not have enough quizzes. Most courses now offer regular quizzes.
4. Some lecture handouts provided no objectives or review questions. The

faculty are slowly updating their handouts, but compliance is not complete.

5. During the first iteration of the new curriculum, students were concerned that the time available to master anatomy was not adequate. The time allotted has remained the same, but the faculty became more comfortable after iteration of the new schedule, and subsequent students were less anxious.

6. Some journal club papers were too long and difficult. We have attempted to correct this problem by asking the directors of each block to nominate at least two candidate papers for each week. The clinical faculty coordinator of the journal club then chooses the most appropriate paper. We still have occasional problems when the basic scientists fail to subject the papers to this approval process.

The students suggested the following modifications of the first-year curriculum:

1. smoothing out of scheduling to achieve consistent pace (this has been done);
2. posting of answer sheets for all problem sets (this has been done);
3. inclusion of patients or their families in all correlation clinics (this has been done);
4. adoption of a consistent policy about posting grades, and returning exams (this has been done);
5. inclusion of objectives, in-text figures, and review questions in all handouts (this has been done for most but not all courses);
6. scheduling of a voluntary review session after each exam (this has been done for some but not all courses);
7. addition of an orientation session for each course (this has been done);
8. provision of more computer learning opportunities (the computer situation is improving);
9. use of frequent, low-stress quizzes throughout the year (this has been done);
10. doubling up of physiology labs to save dogs and improve coordination with lectures (physiology labs have been redesigned to minimize the use of dogs); and
11. an increase in the number of laboratory instructors, so that there are more than two instructors per thirty-five students throughout the year (this has largely been accomplished).

Summary and Conclusions

Our new basic science curriculum is based on a mixture of lectures and discussion groups in which students spend time every day solving problems. This is a form of problem-based learning that differs from the learning offered at many other medical schools because the problems are based on scientific questions, not clinical cases. Nevertheless, virtually every lecture and discussion includes clinical material that illustrates the basic science under discussion. Many discussion and examination questions deal with real or hypothetical patient problems.

We view lectures as necessary because they provide students with the most up-to-date scientific concepts in an efficient manner. We have very high ambitions for our students; we want them to be prepared to do original research, should they choose an academic career. We sought ways to emphasize high-level content delivered in a stimulating, thought-provoking format in order to hold the students' interest. With high-level content, it is impossible for students to organize the material themselves. The lectures emphasize general principles and de-emphasize details, but we try to reach the frontier of scientific knowledge every day. We encourage class participation in lectures, and it is stimulating when this approach works, in the hands of skillful, confident lecturers. However, many faculty prefer to control the lecture hall by suppressing questions.

The first-year committee did not study the curricula or teaching methods at other schools. We were aware of the general philosophy behind problem-based learning as employed elsewhere, but our solution was based on our needs rather than someone else's model. Our changes in the curriculum were largely conservative, built on existing strengths. The new curriculum uses the strongest approaches from the previous courses in all of the new courses.

Some group discussions and examinations require students to have both knowledge of the general principles and the skill to solve problems or propose hypotheses even when no concrete answer is known. These small-group discussions are challenging for faculty members, who must direct the discussion and provide relatively authoritative information on a wide range of topics when discussions expand (as they inevitably do) beyond the prepared questions out to the frontiers of knowledge. After five years, the faculty remain committed to the extra effort.

While our philosophy and the format for the year, the week, and the day have remained constant, the whole curriculum continues to evolve with respect to the details. Each of the first three iterations had a different schedule and a different division of responsibility for the content. All courses have received fine tuning each year in response to student suggestions. Discussion questions change and improve with experience. It is worth noting that the curriculum is relatively robust; it has continued to work well during the past five years as the leadership of most of the courses has changed.

I am impressed with how rapidly small mistakes can lead to general student discontent. The students are so intense and care so much about their education that a misguided comment to the class, a break with a successful routine, a poorly written examination, a long or impossible journal club article, or the failure of a lecturer to know the content of previous talks can upset the students enough to distract them from their usual enthusiasm about biomedical science and their education. Our success lies in having a format that is easy to follow and faculty who are willing to put in the effort to avoid these pitfalls—most of the time.

THE CLINICAL YEARS
Catherine D. De Angelis, M.D.

One of the goals of the new curriculum was to reintroduce the basic sciences into the clinical years. When the index class was in the second year of the new curriculum, a letter was sent to all of the basic science directors asking them (1) to describe their ideas about how this might be accomplished, and (2) to let us know what specific program or programs they might be willing to sponsor. The time period that would be used to teach basic sciences was every other Thursday from 8 to 10 A.M. This period would augment the Physician and Society course that was given on alternate Thursday mornings. The responses were surprisingly positive.

One of the directors suggested that the journal clubs be reintroduced, using more advanced and more directly clinically relevant basic science publications. The small-group format, which was so effective in the first two years, would be used again for this "course." The director of the Department of Biomedical Engineering suggested a course that would cover systems physiology with applications to clinical problems, such as ventricular arrhythmia and hearing aids. Another director suggested a course on the bioscientific aspects of the clinical laboratory.

Rational Therapeutics

After discussing the feasibility issues (i.e., space, faculty time, and student interest), the course that was chosen to be the pilot for the reintroduction of basic sciences in the clinical years was one coordinated by the Department of Pharmacology, called Rational Therapeutics. This course was designed for fourth-year students, on the assumption that they would be thinking about their residencies and eager to review pharmacology. The interactive lecture format was chosen as a trial, and it proved to be very effective because by that time the students were quite accustomed to interaction with faculty presenters. We knew there was a risk of low attendance because so many students would be away due to outside electives, vacations, or interviews for residencies. Therefore, we required only that they attend at least half of the twelve classes to pass the course, which was graded as pass/fail.

At the urging of Dr. Paul Lietman, one of the "Gang of Four" who led the second-year curriculum committee, Dr. Craig Hendrix agreed to direct the course. During the planning period, which lasted a year or so, he met with a number of pharmacology and clinical faculty members who might be willing to participate in the course. Officially the course was offered by the Division of Clinical Pharmacology in the Department of Medicine and by the departments of Pharmacology and of Molecular Biology and Genetics. Each session would involve a pharmacologist and a clinician. The course, as developed, included clinical topics coordinated with pharmacologic principles, as shown in table 3.12.

The course is organized around clinical topics and pharmacologic principles in order to reinforce the use of pharmacologic principles in clinical problem solving regarding the use of drugs. These principles are covered in varying degrees throughout the course as they become pertinent in the drug-related management of a clinical situation. This approach keeps the focus on the clinical situation but reinforces pharmacologic principles. These principles are emphasized in the context of solving therapeutic problems in "real life" situations with which, after more than a year of clinical experience, the students are familiar.

The course requires the generous participation of the pharmacology and clinical faculty working in teams. The format of the course varies with the instructional team, but generally follows the original plan as outlined in our course description. The invited clinical faculty begin with a formal lecture, almost always with slides and some chalkboard work, discussing questions freely as they arise. The first part of the session, the interactive lecture, usually extends well into the second hour due to the active participation of students. The Clinical Pharmacology faculty take the lead in the second hour to ensure that all sequential points in therapeutic decision making are covered, with emphasis on therapeutic monitoring in the very broadest sense. Specifically, how and when does a physician monitor to verify whether and to what degree the chosen therapy achieves the desired therapeutic goal, and what new decisions do these monitoring results necessitate?

Table 3.12   Outline of the Rational Therapeutics Course

Clinical Topics	Pharmacologic Principles
1. Community-acquired pneumonia	1. Clinical pharmacokinetics
2. Angina and coronary artery disease	2. Therapeutic drug monitoring
3. Asthma	3. Adverse drug reactions
4. Anticoagulation	4. Drug allergy
5. Hypertension	5. Drug interactions
6. Congestive heart failure	6. Pharmacogenetics
7. Pain control	7. Dosing in elderly patients
8. Diabetes mellitus	8. Dosing in pediatric patients
9. Shock and ICU issues	9. Dosing in pregnant or lactating women
10. Arthritis and autoimmune disease	10. Dosing in renal and hepatic disease
11. Seizures	11. Substance abuse
12. Peptic ulcer disease	12. Poisoning
	13. Nonprescription drugs
	14. Regulatory issues
	15. Drug development
	16. Writing prescriptions
	17. Learning about new drugs
	18. Selecting among drugs in a therapeutic class
	19. Recognizing pressures to prescribe irrationally

Working through an illustrative case with the class provides an excellent opportunity to reinforce decision-making skills in an interactive context. The presence of several faculty guiding each discussion inevitably leads to the presentation of different approaches to the same clinical problem, but this difference helps to refine the thinking skills of the students as they critically evaluate the faculty when they justify their decisions. Each session provides a healthy mix of educational methods (lecture, discussion, and skills development) appropriate to the educational content.

This course was designed to consolidate student skills in the selection and use of drugs commonly prescribed in medical practice. It is built on the foundation of the second-year Pharmacology course and third-year clinical clerkship experiences. The focus is on therapeutic decision making in the context of clinical problems based on pharmacologic principles. The chosen clinical topics in therapeutics are those that the students will encounter frequently during their residencies. The goal is to stimulate the rational application of core pharmacologic principles that have general applicability to clinical situations throughout a medical career.

The students' and faculty's reactions to the course have been uniformly positive. The two-hour duration of each session is sufficient to cover the topic but not too long. Because of the interactive nature of the course, the students do not become bored. The twice-monthly timing works well because it provides time for the students to use their recently reinforced skills in the clinical settings before coming back for more. The immediate gratification is evident. The students view taking time out from their hectic clinical duties to learn practical clinical problem solving very positively.

One problem that we anticipated was that most of the students were not able to attend all twelve sessions. Therefore, each session was designed to stand on its own. Another issue was raised by the third-year students, who felt neglected because we had planned no special course for their alternate Thursday mornings. Also, the faculty wanted to cover more topics.

Many of these problems and issues were solved by the decision to begin the course in the spring of the third year and end it at the end of the winter session of the fourth year. This allows third-year students to be involved and provides time for more sessions, and therefore allows more topics to be covered. The course was also put on the World Wide Web through the Johns Hopkins InfoNet.

4

The Bridging Sciences

Langford Kidd, M.D., F.R.C.P.,
and Charles M. Wiener, M.D.

The second-year curriculum forms the bridge between the basic sciences in the first year and clinical teaching later, in inpatient and outpatient settings. It introduces students to the disorders of structure and function, and they learn how these disorders produce signs and symptoms in patients and determine the course and outcome of illnesses. Students also study the mechanisms of drug action and encounter the immense and ever-growing armamentarium of medications available to treat disease. Finally, they learn the science and art of history taking and the physical examination. The second year is pivotal in the development of the student into a physician. For many students, it is the first time they must grapple with issues related to professional behavior, such as approaches to death and dying, patient confidentiality, and management of the "difficult" or "uncooperative" patient.

At the outset, it should be made clear that the second year at Johns Hopkins is truncated, comprising only three quarters, each lasting nine weeks. The "year" starts after Labor Day and ends in March at spring break. After spring break, the students return to the Johns Hopkins Medical Institutions and begin their clinical rotations.

The Old Curriculum

The former curriculum, which was instituted in 1967 under the deanship of Dr. David Rogers, involved seven second-year courses (table 4.1).

Pathology

Pathology was a major course that lasted two quarters (eighteen weeks), beginning the day after Labor Day. Pathology instruction introduced the medical stu-

Table 4.1 Duration of Courses in the Old Second-Year Curriculum

Quarter 1		Quarter 2	Quarter 3
Clinical Skills		Clinical Skills	Clinical Skills
Pathology		Pathology	Pharmacology
History of Medicine			Neurology and Neuropathology
Clinical Epidemiology	Human Pathophysiology	Human Pathophysiology	Human Pathophysiology

dent to basic concepts about the mechanisms of disease, stressing alterations in tissues and cells. An overall disease classification was elaborated, and clinical and pathophysiologic correlations were made.

The course started with a brief introduction to general pathology, inflammation, and cellular pathology and then covered immunopathology, microbiology, infectious diseases, and neoplasia. The course then progressed through the various body systems.

In the first quarter, this course was taught every morning, five days a week, with lectures from 9 to 10 A.M. followed by three-hour small-group pathology laboratories. In the second quarter, the frequency decreased to three days a week. The majority of teaching time was devoted to small-group teaching in the pathology laboratories.

There were six small groups of approximately twenty students; each group had as a resource a small, but constant, group of pathology department faculty members, fellows, and residents who were responsible for its instruction throughout the course.

The small-group leaders exercised considerable autonomy regarding what was taught and how the material was presented. This resulted in significant variation among the groups in course material, presentation, and testing. Because of this, a major part of the evaluation was based on the group experience and varied widely across the class. However, one comprehensive, classwide examination was held at the end of the course; in more recent years, it was held before the winter holiday break. In the end, grades were similar among the small groups. Pathology was generally considered to be a strong course, introducing the student to many concepts about disease. The course's perceived strengths included the predominance of small-group teaching and the provision of copious feedback to the students.

Human Pathophysiology

Human Pathophysiology was a major course in the second-year curriculum. In this course the student learned about disordered function and the way in which it produced abnormalities found in the patients whom the students would later encounter in clinical settings. The course was taught throughout the first three quarters of the second year but started three weeks after Pathology, after the brief History of Medicine and Clinical Epidemiology had ended (table 4.1). Human Pathophysiology differed from the Pathology and Pharmacology courses in that it was not a department-based course, but was organized by the dean's office, which appointed a course director, usually from either the Department of Medicine or the Department of Pediatrics. The course was broken up into approximately fifteen sections, each of which dealt with the disorders of function in one of the body systems.

Each individual section was coordinated and planned by a section chief in consultation with the course director and was taught by a varied faculty, of whom 80 percent were from the Department of Medicine and the rest were from the Departments of Pediatrics, Obstetrics and Gynecology, Surgery, and Oncology. The basic model of each class section was a one-hour lecture followed by a two-hour small-group seminar. Most of the seminars took the form of case presentations, which illustrated the points made in the previous lecture, allowed for problem solving, and provided an opportunity for clarification of the lecture material.

There were three Human Pathophysiology examinations—one at the end of each quarter covering the material presented during that quarter. The exams consisted of multiple-choice questions with some brief essays. Students usually evaluated the course favorably; they expressed particular appreciation of the small-group opportunities for case-based learning.

Pharmacology

The Pharmacology course ran for the nine weeks of the third quarter. The objective was to introduce drugs and their actions and interactions. This was basically a lecture course, taught from 9 to 10 A.M. every day, with some workshops and tutorials. It covered the principles of pharmacology, with an emphasis on antibiotics, cardiovascular and renal drugs, endocrine drugs, and central nervous system drugs. In addition, the Pharmacology faculty offered a selection of tutorials that allowed each of the students to select one topic to explore, in depth, in a small-group setting. The course was taught by faculty from the Department of Pharmacology and the Division of Clinical Pharmacology of the Department of

Medicine. Three exams requiring short answers were held during the course. Even though the material to be learned was entirely novel to most students and required much memorization, the course was highly regarded.

History of Medicine

The History of Medicine course extended over nine weeks in the first quarter, with two lectures per week. Its objective was to broaden the background of students; it covered the history of Western medicine from the earliest times to the present day and explored medicine in other cultures. It was taught by members of the Department of History of Medicine. Evaluation was by examination and essay. The course was regarded as interesting and worthwhile, if somewhat academic.

Clinical Epidemiology

The Clinical Epidemiology course consisted of nine three-hour sessions. Held on three afternoons each week, the sessions were made up of a lecture followed by seminar discussions. The course began after Labor Day and ran for three weeks. Its objective was to provide the students with a basic understanding of epidemiologic methods and study design. The students were encouraged to review published medical papers critically and to assess the validity of the papers' experimental designs in order to gain an understanding of the central place of the scientific method in both clinical medicine and clinical investigation. Student achievement was assessed by a series of exercises and a final examination. The course was taught by the Department of Epidemiology of the school of public health and was well regarded.

Neurology and Neuropathology

The Neurology and Neuropathology course was based in the Department of Neurology. Although it was originally designed by Neuropathology faculty, it had developed over the years to encompass a broad spectrum in the pathology and pathophysiology of diseases of the nervous system. The thirty-hour course comprised two three-hour sessions per week for five weeks, each session consisting of a one-hour lecture and two-hour small-group pathology laboratories or discussion groups. Evaluation was based on multiple-choice and brief-answer examinations. This course was well organized and was highly regarded by the students.

Clinical Skills

Clinical Skills was the other major course of the second year. It was taught in three-hour afternoon sessions throughout the year, once per week in the first two quarters and three times per week in the last quarter. There were brief didactic presentations in most weeks, but the course centered on visits to patients by small groups of two to four students, together with one preceptor.

The objective of the course was to provide each student with the opportunity to master the basic skills of history taking and physical examination under the close supervision of a member of the clinical faculty. The students observed and then practiced the techniques of (1) establishing rapport with the patient; (2) obtaining a clinical history; (3) performing a physical examination; (4) presenting this information in both verbal and written forms; and (5) formulating a primary and a differential diagnosis. It was expected that at the end of this course, each student would be prepared for the required clinical clerkships.

The Clinical Skills course dealt with clinical techniques rather than manifestations of disease. During the first two months, instructors remained with students throughout each session to provide immediate feedback and instruction in interviewing techniques and details of the physical examination.

This faculty-intensive course was well organized and was regarded very highly by the students.

Student and Faculty Perspectives

The medical students regarded the old second-year curriculum as good primarily because it was clearly relevant to their long-term goals. The teaching was designed to provide the foundation of knowledge that the students needed to make the transition from basic science in the first year to clinical settings in the fourth quarter of the second year. There were many new vocabulary terms, concepts, and drugs to learn.

The teaching hours were long, running from 9 A.M. to 5 P.M., with only one free afternoon per week. A typical week is illustrated in table 4.2. A highly stressful period for the students was the second quarter (November, December, and January), when the Pathology and Human Pathophysiology teaching became intensive in preparation for the comprehensive final examination in Pathology.

All topics were taught in such a way that their components were dispersed in time and were addressed in the various courses separately. For example, the pathology of the cardiovascular system was taught in October, its pathophysiology was taught in December, and the drugs used in treating cardiovascular disease were taught in March. Some students regarded such repetition as helpful

Table 4.2 Typical Week in the Old Second-Year Curriculum

Time	Monday	Tuesday	Wednesday	Thursday	Friday
9 A.M.–1 P.M.	Pathology, Human Pathophysiology, History of Medicine, or Clinical Epidemiology	Pathology	Human Pathophysiology Clinicopathologic Conference	Pathology	Pathology
2–5 P.M.	Clinical Skills	Human Pathophysiology and Clinical Skills	Free	Human Pathophysiology and Clinical Skills	Human Pathophysiology or Neuropathology

and reinforcing, allowing for revisiting of material previously studied, while others considered it to be duplicative, disorganized, and not conducive to systematic learning.

Because the courses were separate units, there was little or no consultation between the faculty who taught them. Dissonance and contradiction between courses could and often did occur. Further, examinations often disrupted teaching: students would skip class in one course to prepare for an exam in another.

The faculty regarded the second year as a good teaching experience. The teaching of Pathology and Pharmacology was circumscribed; these classes occupied only two quarters and one quarter, respectively, and occurred at the same time each day. They were departmentally based, and the time and effort expended on them by the faculty were valued and recognized by the respective chairs. The considerable efforts of the thirty faculty members in the Clinical Skills course, many of them teaching part-time, were also reported to their departmental chairs. The Human Pathophysiology faculty enjoyed the luxury of teaching in short time periods because each subspecialty group was involved for only a one- or two-week period annually.

Planning the Second-Year Curriculum

The Gang of Four

Early in 1992, Dr. Catherine De Angelis, vice dean for academic affairs, appointed Dr. Langford Kidd to be coordinator of the second-year curriculum. He had previously worked with her on the coordination of the Human Pathophysiology course. His first step in revising the second-year curriculum was to meet with the directors of the departments of Pharmacology and Pathology and with the course directors of Pharmacology, Pathology, and Clinical Skills to set up a working group. Soon known as the "Gang of Four," the working group consisted of the course directors of Pharmacology (Dr. Paul Lietman), Pathology (Dr. Jean Olson), Clinical Skills (Dr. Lawrence Griffith), and Human Pathophysiology (Dr. Langford Kidd). Their mission was to discuss, plan, develop, and implement the new second-year curriculum. In the planning stage the Gang of Four met for two to three hours weekly, beginning with an off-campus retreat and continuing with on-campus meetings. After much discussion, it was decided to persevere with the model of medical school teaching traditional to Johns Hopkins—that is, a mixture of lectures and small-group teaching. However, there would be an increased emphasis on small-group discussion sections in a nonlecture format and a decreased number of large-group lectures. The discussion sections would be oriented toward case-based problem solving (ex. 4.1) and led by mem-

Example 4.1   Case-Based Problem

A young woman, previously healthy, develops a neurologic disorder—Guillain-Barré syndrome, which causes ascending paralysis that can involve respiratory muscles. As a pulmonary consultant, you are asked to evaluate her. She has severe weakness of the legs and moderate weakness of the arms. She has no weakness of the head or neck muscles and has a normal gag reflex and normal swallowing. She denies any shortness of breath. You make the following measurements:

Arterial Blood Gases

	Actual	Normal
PO_2	90	(80–100)
PCO_2	43	(35–45)
pH	7.43	(7.35–7.45)
	Actual	Predicted
Minute ventilation	7 L/min	(5–10)
Tidal volume	0.5 L	(0.5)
Vital capacity	1 L	(4 L)
FEV_1	0.8 L	(3.2 L)
Maximum voluntary ventilation	15 L/min	(112 L/min)

What would you recommend?

Assume that the patient's CO_2 production is 200 ml/min. What is the arterial PCO_2 for the following levels of alveolar ventilation?

Hint: $P_aCO_2 = 0.863 \times \dot{V}CO_2 \text{ (ml/min)} \div \dot{V}_A \text{ (L/min)}$

V_A (L/min)	P_aCO_2 (mm Hg)
1	
2	
4	
8	

Plot these results.

Answer: The arterial blood gases are normal. The minute ventilation is normal, and the normal arterial carbon dioxide indicates adequate alveolar ventilation. The reduction in vital capacity is severe, as is the reduction in maximum voluntary ventilation, which should be about 40 times the FEV_1.

Sustaining a minute ventilation in excess of 50 percent of maximum ventilation will rapidly lead to respiratory muscle fatigue in most individuals. If fatigue occurs, the patient will be unable to sustain her basal ventilation, and alveolar hypoventilation, hypercapnia, and hypoxemia will ensue. Respiratory muscle function will be fur-

(*continued*)

Example 4.1   (*continued*)

ther impaired by the blood gas abnormalities; alveolar ventilation will be further impaired by the rapid shallow breathing pattern of fatigue; and the blood gas abnormalities will worsen as the muscle function deteriorates.

Because of the hyperbolic relationship of arterial PCO_2 to alveolar ventilation, small decreases in ventilation can lead to large increases in hypercapnia. See the graph below, which plots the alveolar ventilation equation, assuming a normal production of 200 ml/min of CO_2.

Because this individual is at high risk for a spiraling downward course of respiratory failure leading to respiratory arrest and death, she is at grave risk. She should be closely monitored with respect to arterial blood gases, and should be mechanically ventilated at the first signs of respiratory failure. If adequate monitoring facilities are not available, then it would be prudent to prophylactically put this subject on mechanical ventilation. Measure to improve the underlying condition should also be undertaken, of course.

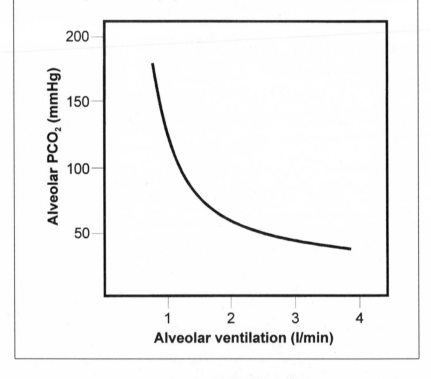

bers of the faculty. A switch to a problem-based learning curriculum was discussed but not recommended for adoption because it was perceived as (1) requiring a prolonged start-up period before implementation; (2) difficult to introduce to students with no previous exposure; (3) extremely labor intensive for the faculty; and (4) not necessarily in the best interest of students. The outcomes of this approach had not been demonstrated to differ significantly from the outcomes of more traditional methods of learning, including case-based learning.

The Basic Concept

The basic concept for second-year teaching was that we should coordinate, and to a certain extent integrate, the teaching in the main courses—Pathology, Human Pathophysiology, and Pharmacology—and that these subjects should be taught together rather than separately. That is, we would use an organ-systems-based approach to teaching. Instruction about the heart and circulation, for example, would be planned so as to allow the students to learn the pathophysiology of heart failure, the pathology of heart failure, and the drugs used to treat heart failure, all at the same time. This organization would encourage students to learn in an integrated, elaborated way, rather than in the previously used, more linear manner, in which integration of the whole picture often had to wait until the clinical years. The Pathology, Human Pathophysiology, and Pharmacology courses would form the "core curriculum" of the second year.

The fourth major course was Clinical Skills. This course was planned to continue its afternoon sessions in the hope that it could also be coordinated with the core curriculum. The Physician and Society course (chap. 5) would also continue throughout the second year.

These changes meant that two of the courses previously taught in the second year, History of Medicine and Clinical Epidemiology, would be moved to the first year. The History of Medicine course became part of the Physician and Society course, and Clinical Epidemiology was taught as a separate course in the first-year curriculum. The Neurology and Neuropathology course became part of the organ-systems-based core curriculum in the second year instead of being taught as a separate course in the first year. Thus, it was decided that there would be five courses in the second year—Pathology, Human Pathophysiology, Pharmacology, Clinical Skills, and Physician and Society—and, therefore, that five grades would be given at the end of that year.

Integration and Coordination

When the Gang of Four and the vice dean held discussions with the directors of the departments of Pathology and Pharmacology and the directors of the Pathology and Pharmacology courses, it was agreed that coordination of the teaching in the core curriculum was desirable. However, there were strong feelings that departmental autonomy should be preserved and that there was great virtue in having Pathology taught by pathologists and Pharmacology taught by pharmacologists.

Therefore, we decided to move forward in our second-year planning with coordination and some degree of integration, but without abandoning or blurring the margins of the individual disciplines. It was agreed that teaching in the various areas should be planned jointly, with interdepartmental consultation, but that each lecture or small-group session should be clearly identified as belonging to Pathology, Pharmacology, or Human Pathophysiology. It was hoped that conjoint sessions would be developed, and this has occurred over the years. However, it will take more time for the vestiges of departmental chauvinism to disappear completely.

The Emphasis on Case Orientation and Small-Group Teaching

Small-group teaching was already a strong feature of the second-year curriculum and had been used extensively in the Pathology laboratories and in the case-study seminars of the Human Pathophysiology course. It was the norm in the Clinical Skills course, in which two to four students met with one preceptor at the patient's side. Small-group teaching in the Pharmacology course took the form of tutorials.

We decided to emphasize that the small-group teaching should not consist of mini-lectures but should be case-oriented and devoted to developing problem-solving skills. We also increased the number of small-group sessions and reduced the number of lectures. We had experimented with the nonlecture format in the Lung section of the Human Pathophysiology course. Despite the increased demands on their time, the faculty responsible for the Lung Section enjoyed this teaching style, and more of them had the opportunity to interact closely with students. However, the students felt insecure without the maps and signposts supplied by the lectures, and this course of action was abandoned. On average, a mix of 50 percent lectures and 50 percent small-group sessions seemed to work well for the students.

Increasing Time for Independent Study

We decided to reduce the hours of classroom time, where possible, so that more time could be devoted to self-directed learning and independent study. This was a difficult task with so much material to cover in such a short time, especially since we had moved several topics from the first year to the second year.

When the first- and second-year planners reviewed the curriculum as a whole, we found that in the old curriculum, Psychiatry and Behavioral Sciences had been taught as an independent course toward the end of the first year, before students had any exposure to other aspects of disease. We decided that this course should be taught during the second year. Another major topic of discussion was the teaching of Microbiology, which had been part of the first-year curriculum. Both students and faculty complained that the first-year teaching on the basic science aspects of microbiology did little to prepare students for the study of organisms pathogenic to humans in the second-year Infectious Diseases section. So discussions were held with the first-year faculty to change the teaching of Microbiology in year 1, in the hope that it could be expanded and made more medically relevant. This did not occur, so the teaching time for Infectious Diseases in the second year was dramatically increased and basic microbiology was incorporated into that section.

We were able to accommodate these additions to the second-year curriculum by moving Clinical Epidemiology to the first year and incorporating History of Medicine into the first-year Physician and Society course. By compressing some second-year material and beginning classes one hour earlier each day, we were able to allow two free afternoons per week in the first quarter. One of these afternoons was filled by Clinical Skills in the second quarter.

The New Second-Year Curriculum

After the entire second-year curriculum was reviewed, we identified teaching deficiencies in areas such as the musculoskeletal system, rheumatology, reproduction, and the eye. Areas of overlap were identified and eliminated. For example, we decided that systemic hypertension should be taught only by the kidney group rather than by both that group and the heart and circulation group. We also decided to add a Growth, Development, and Aging section to draw attention to the variations in disease patterns and drug sensitivities at the two extremes of life. A section on human sexuality, a subject perceived as having been somewhat neglected previously, was also added.

We decided to divide the second-year curriculum into two modules: an introductory module, which contained teaching of material common to many of the systems, and an organ system module. It was estimated that the first module would consist of 169 hours and cover six weeks, and that the second would consist of 450 hours and cover twenty-one weeks (table 4.3).

The individual sections were planned to be taught separately and in succession, except for two groupings: Introduction to Pathology would be paired with Introduction to Pharmacology, and Neurology and Neuropathology would be integrated with Psychiatry and Behavioral Sciences. These two double sections were to be taught simultaneously. Each curricular unit was identified as belonging to Pathology, Human Pathophysiology, or Pharmacology. To aid in identifi-

Table 4.3   Modules and Sections in the New Second-Year Curriculum

Introductory Module		Organ System Module	
Section	Hours	Section	Hours
Introduction to Pathology	14	Liver and Gastrointestinal Tract	59
Introduction to Pharmacology	14	Eye	10
Neoplasia	23	Skin	14
Genetics	3	Psychiatry and Behavioral Sciences	52
Immunology	25	Neurology and Neuropathology	55
Growth, Development, and Aging	19	Heart and Circulation	47
Infectious Diseases	64	Kidney	41
Nutrition	7	Lung	35
		Human Sexuality	19
		Reproduction	34
		Endocrine	26
		Blood	32
		Bone and Connective Tissue	26

cation, Pathology handouts were reproduced on white paper, Human Patho-physiology on pink, and Pharmacology on blue.

The Schedule

We resolved that each day's core curriculum teaching would start at 8 A.M., one hour earlier than second-year teaching had begun previously, and that teaching would continue until lunchtime at 1 P.M. The core curriculum would also be taught two afternoons per week in the first two quarters, and Clinical Skills would be taught one afternoon per week during the same period, leaving two free afternoons for independent study. In the third quarter, when Clinical Skills expanded to three afternoons per week, core curriculum teaching was reduced to one afternoon, leaving one free afternoon per week. Physician and Society was taught on Thursdays from 11 A.M. to 1 P.M. (table 4.4).

Coordination of Courses

Originally, we had hoped to coordinate the content of Clinical Skills with what was being taught simultaneously in the core curriculum. For example, we hoped that instruction on the heart and circulation would coincide with instruction on the physical examination of the cardiovascular system and its assessment in health

Table 4.4 Typical Week in the New Second-Year Curriculum, 1993/94 (First Iteration)

Time	Monday	Tuesday	Wednesday	Thursday	Friday
8 A.M.	Alkylating Agents (PH)	Bacterial Structure and Virulence (P)	Bacterial Physiology (P)	Gram Negative Bacteria (P)	Pathology of Bacterial Diseases (P)
9 A.M.	Tumor Progression and Cell Heterogeneity (PP)	Small group (P)	Small group (P)	Small group (P)	Small group (P)
10 A.M.	Small group case presentations (PP)				
11 A.M.		Sulfonamides and Antifolates (PH)	Penicillins and Cephalosporins I (PH)	Physician and Society (PAS)	Erythromycin, Clindamycin, Chloramphenicol, Tetracyclines (PH)
12 noon	Resistance to Antineoplastic Agents (PH)	Lunch	Penicillins and Cephalosporins II (PH)		Lunch
1 P.M.	Lunch	Gram Positive Bacteria (PH)	Lunch	Free	Sexually Transmitted Diseases (PP)
2 P.M.	Physical Examination (CS)	Small Group (P)	Free	Free	Small Group (P)
3 P.M.	Small group		Free	Free	Free
4 P.M.	Free	Free	Free	Free	

Note: CS = Clinical Skills; P = Pathology; PAS = Physician and Society; PH = Pharmacology; PP = Human Pathophysiology.

and disease. However, this hope proved to be elusive. The first part of Clinical Skills was devoted to the mastery of history taking and the normal physical examination. This had no counterpart in the organ-based core curriculum, which meant that a considerable portion of the core curriculum would elapse before it was possible to focus on organ-based teaching in the Clinical Skills course. A second factor that made classroom–bedside coordination difficult was that when a section in a given subject area was being taught from 8 A.M. to 1 P.M. five days per week, it was difficult to find a large number of specialists in that area to teach clinical skills in the afternoons. This would have left them no time for other duties.

Since the content of the Physician and Society course was planned to relate to the entire four years, many of the curricular objectives of the course were separate and distinct from the second-year core curriculum. However, the Physician and Society course has evolved to cover more topics that are related to the core curriculum and that are compatible philosophically with the "bridging" nature of the second year. Topics such as "The Physician and the Pharmaceutical Industry" and "Interviewing the Homosexual Patient" enable students to examine the complex issues that are part of the everyday life of a clinician. The Physician and Society course is discussed in chapter 5.

Computers and Informatics

One of the objectives of basic science education in the new curriculum was to encourage the students to review current literature critically and insightfully. Therefore, each student was required to take a practicum in literature searching and retrieval in the first year. Many sources of second-year material were made available through the computers in the Welch Medical Library and in the Preclinical Teaching Building. Students could review old exam questions on-line and use commercial CD-ROM-based programs. In the second and third iterations of the curriculum, more and more lecture articles and handouts, as well as old examinations, became available. As the core curriculum took shape, plans were made to include as much material as possible on the LectureLinks network, described in chapter 6. Currently, images from Pathology, lectures from Human Pathophysiology, and old examinations from the three core courses are available on LectureLinks.

The Focus Groups

The Gang of Four appointed a focus group for each section, made up of faculty members for that section, to be responsible for the detailed planning of teaching in the section. Each focus group consisted of a pathologist, a pharmacologist, and a pathophysiologist familiar with each organ system and other experts if needed. For example, a cardiac electrophysiologist and a pediatric cardiologist were added to the focus group for the Heart and Circulation section.

We selected a leader for each focus group, and each group was then invited to meet with the Gang of Four to discuss the proposed changes in the curriculum. The focus groups held meetings with the appropriate faculty to discuss the coordination of teaching in their particular areas with the core curriculum overall and to develop proposals for their time blocks. Each proposal was reviewed by the focus groups and the Gang of Four, and any areas of overlap or imbalance were identified. Only then was the final plan prepared.

We developed a schedule for the various subjects, determined the duration of each section, and spaced the exams. It was decided that seven coordinated examinations would be held at intervals throughout the year, each one focusing on the material covered in all areas during the previous three to four weeks, and that each exam would have clearly identified sections belonging to Pathology, Human Pathophysiology, and/or Pharmacology. In accordance with these policies, exams are now given on Monday mornings or just before holidays. Exams begin at 8:30 A.M. with a twenty-minute pathology laboratory quiz involving glass slides or Kodachromes. From 9 A.M. to 1 P.M., students take separate Pathology, Human Pathophysiology, and Pharmacology examinations. The course directors coordinate the sizes of their individual exams so that the expected duration of the total examination is three hours (with another hour available for students who need it). Students are given all three exams at once so that they can allocate their time individually. Currently, the exams are not cross-disciplinary. One goal for the future is developing a cross-disciplinary comprehensive final examination and, possibly, making the seven coordinated exams cross-disciplinary as well.

Each focus group was responsible for recruiting the faculty, including lecturers and instructors, for the small-group sessions. The focus groups met with the lecturers to decide what subject matter should be covered in the sessions. They also met with the small-group teachers to make sure they knew what material, usually case-based problem solving, was to be covered in each of the small-group sessions or in the Pathology laboratories. All faculty involved in a section were encouraged to attend all of the lectures during that section in order to be familiar with the material being presented outside their areas.

The New Curriculum in Practice

One of Dr. Kidd's most important roles was to monitor the progress of the new curriculum in practice. By attending most of the lectures throughout the year, he was able to meet with the focus group leaders and the students on an informal day-to-day basis. This allowed for midcourse modifications and readjustments. The Gang of Four met weekly throughout the year to check on progress, evaluate the various sections, set the structure of the exams (determining the time allotted to each course), and discuss student problems.

Each second-year class elected a Student Education Committee, which met with Dr. Kidd and/or the Gang of Four on various occasions to discuss perceived problems and to engage in bi-directional feedback. In general, these meetings were considered worthwhile by both the students and the faculty.

From the student perspective, a major problem in the first iteration of the new second-year curriculum was the distinct change of pace between year 1 and year 2. In year 1, teaching was confined to the mornings, and the atmosphere was that of a graduate school, with an informal approach to learning. There were few concentrated parts of the curriculum. The number of faculty who taught the courses was smaller than in the second year, and the students and faculty all knew each other.

In year 2, however, the teaching was much more concentrated and time-consuming. The students had to learn many new terms and concepts of disease and drug action. The faculty was entirely new to the students, and each faculty group made a relatively brief appearance before being replaced by another group covering another topic. The pace was faster than in year 1, and the exams were perceived as being more threatening. While the new curriculum increased the time available for independent study in the second year by more than 100 percent, most afternoons were still full. The small-group sessions were often mini-lectures used to present new material and were seldom either reflective or student-directed.

The greater difficulty of year 2 sometimes made conceptual coordination impractical. For example, it seemed logical, pedagogically, to link the teaching of the heart, kidney, and lungs together in one block, as a conceptually cohesive unit. However, the vast amount of new content and material in this section was perceived as extraordinarily heavy, and the students' mastery of it was tested in a single examination on the three organ systems. This proved to be very stressful for the students.

As the year progressed, however, and the students grew more accustomed to the change of pace, their discomfort was ameliorated, and a more balanced view prevailed. Students enjoyed the emphasis on disease and therapeutics because it seemed more relevant to their futures as physicians. What had happened, in fact, was that the trauma of the conventional first year of medical school had been transferred to the second year, and the students had not been prepared for it.

In general, the students appreciated the coordination between the three constituents of the core curriculum, and they questioned why the Clinical Skills course could not be better coordinated with the others. We invited interested students to help us plan for such coordination, but thus far, no workable plan has emerged.

From the faculty perspective, the main issue was changes in the structure of the teaching sessions. Previously, teaching had started at 9 A.M., but it now began at 8 A.M. In the old curriculum, the Pathology, Human Pathophysiology, and Pharmacology faculty had been accustomed to teaching at certain hours on certain days of each week and could plan their other functions around these times. In the new curriculum, teaching began earlier and there were no regular times for the teaching of Pathology, Pathophysiology, or Pharmacology because the flow of teaching was dictated by the need to coordinate subject matter. For instance, teaching about antiarrhythmic drugs followed teaching about arrhythmias and could occur at any time during the morning.

Basically, however, despite some discomfort with change, there was a general appreciation that the coordination between the teaching of the three major subjects produced a more cohesive and meaningful curriculum. There are still a few instances of lack of communication, and we continue to work on this.

Modifications

In summary, as a result of what we learned from the first class that completed the second-year curriculum, we decided to

1. increase still further the amount of time for independent study;
2. present the entire core curriculum during the mornings;
3. increase the time scheduled for the teaching of the Microbiology and Infectious Diseases sections;
4. improve the teaching in individual sections; and
5. avoid undue congestion in any part of the curriculum.

To achieve these aims, we made a number of modifications. The Nutrition section was moved back to the first year, and an independent Genetics course was eliminated because genetics teaching permeated the whole of the second-year curriculum. The Growth, Development, and Aging course was dropped because most of the material it covered was also covered in other courses. The teaching of human sexuality, which had been juxtaposed with the teaching of reproduction, was included in the Psychiatry and Behavioral Sciences section. The Heart and Circulation section and the Lung section were taught in juxtaposition, and the Kidney section was moved to decongest that part of the schedule. To clear the afternoons and further rationalize the curriculum, the Physician and Society course was shifted from morning to afternoon.

These changes allowed the core curriculum to be taught between 8 A.M. and 1 P.M. five days a week (table 4.5). The only activities in the afternoon were Clinical Skills, which was taught one afternoon a week in the first two quarters and three afternoons a week in the third quarter, and Physician and Society. Elective Pharmacology tutorials, which provided an opportunity for the students to meet with a pharmacologist and discuss a single topic in depth, also took place on the unscheduled afternoons throughout the year.

The second iteration of the new curriculum was received with much more appreciation by students, who perhaps had been prepared for the change of pace between year 1 and year 2 by the class that had gone before. The Heart and Circulation section and the Lung section were still considered a difficult block, but in general, student acceptance increased markedly.

The teaching of Infectious Diseases continued to be a problem. It had proved impossible to develop appropriate coverage of microorganisms pathogenic to humans in the first-year Microbiology course; therefore, a major expansion of this section in the second year was a high priority. To provide sufficient time for the expansion, a week was added to the end of the second-year Microbiology and Infectious Diseases section. This week previously had been devoted to a mini-course entitled Advanced Clinical Skills, which was no longer relevant.

In the third iteration of the new second-year curriculum, the radically redesigned teaching of Microbiology and Infectious Diseases was well received. The Heart and Circulation section and the Kidney section were taught as one block, and the combination was still perceived as too heavy; therefore, Heart and Circulation, Lung, and Kidney were completely separated from one another in the fourth iteration. The schedule for the fourth iteration is illustrated in table 4.6.

The Current Curriculum

The Gang of Four became the Gang of Five when the director of the Physician and Society course, Dr. Leon Gordis, joined the group. In 1996 Dr. Kidd retired, and Dr. Charles Wiener became the director of the Human Pathophysiology course and leader of the Gang of Five. Each year the five meet with the focus groups to discuss the feedback from students and the concerns of all faculty members about their parts of the curriculum. For each course the teaching and faculty are reviewed and the focus group produces a revised plan for the next year and presents it to the Gang of Five.

Table 4.5 Typical Week in the New Second-Year Curriculum, 1995/96 (Third Iteration)

Time	Monday	Tuesday	Wednesday	Thursday	Friday
8 A.M.	Left Ventricular Function (PP)	Cardiomyopathies (PP)	Parasympathetic Drugs (PH)	Inotropic Drugs II (PH)	Nitrates (PH)
9 A.M.	Acute and Chronic Changes in Cardiac Failure (PP)	Myocardial, Biochemical, and Systematic Abnormalities in Heart Failure (PP)	Sympathetic Drugs (PH)	Cardiovascular Pharmacokinetics (PH)	Pediatric Congenital Heart Disease (PP)
10 A.M.	Cardiomyopathy (P)	Seminar: Heart Failure I (PP)	Seminar: Heart Failure II (PP)	Journal Club: Congestive Heart Failure (PP/PH)	
11 A.M.	Small group: Pathology of Congestive Heart Failure (P)				Seminar/lab: Pediatric Cardiology (P/PP)
12 noon		ACE Inhibitors (PH)	Inotropic Drugs I (PH)	Calcium Channel Blockers and Beta Blockers (PH)	
1 P.M.	Free	Lunch	Lunch	Free	Free
2 P.M.	Free	Physician and Society: Selective II (PAS)	Small group/lab: Phlebotomy Techniques (CS)	Free	Free
3 P.M.	Free			Free	Free
4 P.M.	Free	Free		Free	Free

Note: CS = Clinical Skills; P = Pathology; PAS = Physician and Society; PH = Pharmacology; PP = Human Pathophysiology.

Table 4.6   1996/97 Schedule of the Second-Year Curriculum

Week	Monday	Tuesday	Wednesday	Thursday	Friday
09/02/96	Holiday	Regist/Intro	Intro P/PH	Intro P/PH	Intro P/PH
09/09/96	Intro P/PH	Neoplasia	Neoplasia	Neoplasia	Neoplasia
09/16/96	Neoplasia	Blood	Blood	Blood	Blood
09/23/96	Study day	Blood	Blood	Blood	Immuno
09/30/96	Immuno	Immuno	Immuno/Rheum	Rheum	Rheum
10/07/96	Exam 1	ID	ID	ID	ID
10/14/96	ID	ID	ID	ID	ID
10/21/96	ID	ID	ID	ID	ID
10/28/96	ID	ID	ID	ID	ID
11/04/96	Exam 2	Endocrine	Endocrine	Endocrine	Endocrine
11/11/96	Endocrine	Kidney	Kidney	Kidney	Kidney
11/18/96	Kidney	Kidney	Kidney	Kidney	Kidney
11/25/96	Exam 3	Heart	Heart	Holiday	Holiday
12/02/96	Heart	Heart	Heart	Heart	Heart
12/09/96	Heart	Heart	Heart	Bone	Bone
12/16/96	Bone	Skin	Skin	Skin	Exam 4
12/23/96	Winter break	Winter break	Winter break	Winter break	Winter break
12/30/96	Winter break	Winter break	Winter break	Eye	Eye
01/06/97	Liver	Liver	Liver	GI	GI
01/13/97	GI	GI	GI	GI	GI
01/20/97	Holiday	Exam 5	Lung	Lung	Lung
01/27/97	Lung	Lung	Lung	Lung	Reprod
02/03/97	Reprod	Reprod	Reprod	Reprod	Reprod
02/10/97	Exam 6	PS/N/HS	PS/N/HS	PS/N/HS	PS/N/HS
02/17/97	Holiday	PS/N/HS	PS/N/HS	PS/N/HS	PS/N/HS
02/24/97	PS/N/HS	PS/N/HS	PS/N/HS	PS/N/HS	PS/N/HS
03/03/97	PS/N/HS	PS/N/HS	PS/N/HS	PS/N/HS	PS/N/HS
03/10/97	PS/N/HS	PS/N/HS	PS/N/HS	PS/N/HS	PS/N/HS
03/17/97	PS/N/HS	PS/N/HS	PS/N/HS	PS/N/HS	Exam 7
03/24/97	Spring break	Spring break	Spring break	Spring break	Spring break

Note: GI = Gastrointestinal Tract; Heart = Heart and Circulation; HS = Human Sexuality; ID = Infectious Diseases; Immuno = Immunology; N = Neurology and Neuropathology; P = Pathology; PH = Pharmacology; PS = Psychiatry and Behavioral Science; Reprod = Reproduction; Rheum = Rheumatology.

The process of curricular change at Johns Hopkins is still evolving, and the second-year curriculum is no exception. While the change was initiated centrally, the redesigned second-year curriculum represented the deliberations of more than a hundred members of focus groups and other faculty. The departments of Pathology and Pharmacology surrendered some of their autonomy in teaching their own courses so that the curriculum could be coordinated and become an integral whole. To some extent, integration has occurred, and the instances of integrated presentations are growing. Multidisciplinary small-group sessions (e.g., Breast Cancer) have been developed and are viewed as successful by faculty and students. The integrated small-group sessions in the Infectious Diseases section, in which a pathologist, a pathophysiologist (usually a member of the Infectious Diseases faculty), and a clinical pharmacologist discuss case studies with students, have been outstanding (ex. 4.2). Progress is taking place in other areas toward making integration part of the accepted mind-set and removing the remaining departmental barriers.

Currently, the initial portion of the core curriculum consists of four days of Introduction to Pharmacology and Pathology, five days of Neoplasia, three days of Immunology, nineteen days of Microbiology and Infectious Diseases, and seven days of Blood. Introduction to Pharmacology and Pathology, which emphasizes principles that are necessary for moving into the organ-specific sections, includes lectures and small groups addressing pharmacokinetics, drug design and development, inflammation, and cell death.

The Microbiology and Infectious Diseases section was placed immediately after Introduction to Pharmacology and Pathology because the faculty felt that it laid a foundation essential to subsequent organ-system-based learning. This is especially true because the Microbiology and Infectious Diseases section concurrently teaches basic microbiology (a traditional first-year subject), as well as human pathophysiology and therapeutics (traditional second-year subjects). The section is divided into subsections on bacteria, viruses, fungi, and parasites. There is excellent integration between the courses: the antimicrobials relevant to each class of microbe are introduced after presentation of the microbes and their pathophysiology, and multidisciplinary case discussions take place at the end of each subsection. Students in previous years were distressed by the partial "first year" tone of the Microbiology section, but liked learning the clinical applications simultaneously. Informing the students that the Microbiology and Infectious Diseases section is a hybrid combining traditional first-year and second-year material, and moving it to the early portion of year 2 before the students have had much clinical exposure, has lessened this distress.

In the Blood section, which follows Microbiology and Infectious Diseases, students learn about the normal and abnormal formation of red blood cells, of white blood cells, of platelets, and of the coagulation cascade taught in Pathology and Human Pathophysiology. In Pharmacology there are lectures on anticoagulants and antiplatelet agents. After completion of the initial eight weeks of instruction, the students are well prepared to proceed with the remaining nineteen weeks of organ-system-based sections. The schedule of the sections is based on pedagogical principles allowing for practical modifications (table 4.7). Areas

---

Example 4.2   Multidisciplinary Case Discussion Guide

A 40-year-old business executive traveled in Africa, May 17–26. The nurse at the company clinic suggested he take malaria chemoprophylaxis. He declined, believing he would not be in an endemic area. His business took him to Nairobi, Kenya, where he spent most of the week. An unexpected break in his schedule allowed him to travel to one of the nearby game parks, where he spent the night.

Ten days after his return to Baltimore on June 5, he awoke with fever, chills, a dry cough, and a headache. He saw his personal physician, who prescribed erythromycin. He took his medication but felt increasingly ill, and two days later went to a local hospital emergency room.

There he had a fever of 104.2° Fahrenheit and appeared quite ill. His physical examination was remarkable for a palpable spleen tip in the left upper quadrant, diminished deep tendon reflexes, and pupils sluggishly reactive to light. Lab tests revealed a hemoglobin of 7.8 gm/dL (normal 13–16); hematocrit 28% (nl 41–45); white blood count of 4,400/mm^3 (nl 4,500–9,000); platelets 36,000/mm^3 (nl 150,000–350,000); alanine aminotransferase 88 units/mL (nl 8–40); total bilirubin 3.4 mg/dL (nl < 1.2). A blood smear was obtained that revealed the diagnosis.

The emergency room physician recommended admission, but the hospital was full. The patient was sent home and told to return in the morning. At home, later that night, the patient became increasingly unresponsive. He suffered a grand mal seizure and his wife called an ambulance. He was admitted to the hospital intensive care unit, where despite appropriate therapy, he suffered continued neurological deterioration and died on the fourth hospital day.

What is the diagnosis?

Is it important to make a precise diagnosis from the blood smear? How would this change your recommended treatment?

What would have been appropriate therapy for this patient?

Could this disease have been prevented? How?

Key Characteristics of Case 11

Pathophysiology/ID

1. Always take a travel history.
2. Severe malaria (= ICU)
   Abnormal level of consciousness, > 3% parasitemia, Hct < 20%, hypo-

(continued)

Example 4.2 (*continued*)

glycemia, renal/hepatic/cardiovascular/pulmonary dysfunction, DIC, severe vomiting/diarrhea, prolonged hypothermia.
3. Hypoglycemia is common and probably due both to the parasite and to quinine therapy (induction of insulin release).
4. If suspected: thick and thin smears every 8–12 hours for 3 days.
5. Progression can be quite rapid in the non-immune.

Microbiology

For diagnosis a blood specimen should be received in the laboratory within 2 hours of collection, and these are accepted by the laboratory anytime (24 hours).

Thin smears are necessary for speciation, and results are normally available 2 hours after receipt of the specimens. Thick smears (which increase sensitivity) require 8–12 hours for results to be completed.

It is recommended that initial specimens be drawn immediately if malaria is suspected; it is not necessary to wait for fever spike. If first specimen is negative, additional samples may be submitted for examination at approximately 8–12 hour intervals, or 2–3 hours after fever spike for 3 days.

If *Plasmodium falciparum* is identified, an estimate of the number of erythrocytes parasitized should be performed.

Pharmacology

All *falciparum* malaria (especially with cerebral involvement) is potentially life-threatening and requires prompt treatment. For severe disease, use parenteral quinine (if available) or quinidine. For less severe disease, use mefloquine, or quinine plus fansidar, or quinine plus a tetracycline antibiotic.

Assume all malaria is *falciparum* until proven otherwise. Assume all *falciparum* is chloroquine-resistant unless you and the patient are absolutely certain the malaria was acquired in one of the few areas where chloroquine-sensitive *falciparum* still exists.

It is important to speciate malaria from a thin smear if possible, since virtually all non-*falciparum* species can be treated with chloroquine (the exception is a small pocket of chloroquine-resistant *ovale* in the South Pacific).

Primaquine treatment is indicated for non-*falciparum* malaria to eradicate liver stages.

Table 4.7   1997/98 Schedule of the Second-Year Curriculum

Week	Monday	Tuesday	Wednesday	Thursday	Friday
09/01/97	Holiday	Regist/Orient	Intro	Intro	Intro
09/08/97	Intro	Neoplasia	Neoplasia	Neoplasia	Neoplasia
09/15/97	Neoplasia	Immuno	Immuno	Immuno	Immuno
09/22/97	Exam 1	ID	ID	ID/ID	ID
09/29/97	ID	ID	ID	Reading day	ID
10/06/97	ID	ID	ID	ID	ID/CPC
10/13/97	ID	ID	ID	ID/ID	ID
10/20/97	Exam 2	Free day	Blood	Blood/Blood	Blood/Blood
10/27/97	Blood	Blood	Blood	Rheum/Rheum	Rheum
11/03/97	Rheum	Lung	Lung	Lung/Lung	Lung/CPC
11/10/97	Lung	Lung	Lung	Eye	Eye
11/17/97	Exam 3	Renal	Renal	Renal/Renal	Renal
11/24/97	Renal	Renal	Renal	Holiday	Holiday
12/01/97	Renal	Renal	Heart	Heart/Heart	Heart/CPC
12/08/97	Heart	Heart	Heart	Heart/Heart	Heart
12/15/97	Exam 4	Liver	Liver	Liver/Liver	Liver
01/05/98	GI	GI	GI	GI	GI/PH I
01/12/98	GI	GI	Skin	Skin	Skin/CPC/PH II
01/19/98	Holiday	Endocrine	Endocrine	Endocrine	Endocrine
01/26/98	Endocrine	Reprod	Reprod	Reprod	Reprod PH III
02/02/98	Reprod	Reprod	Bone	Bone	Bone/CPC/PH IV
02/09/98	Exam 5	Psych/Neuro	Psych/Neuro	Psych/Neuro	Psych/Neuro
02/16/98	Holiday	Psych/Neuro	Psych/Neuro	Psych/Neuro	Psych/Neuro
02/23/98	Psych/Neuro	Psych/Neuro	Psych/Neuro	Psych/Neuro	Psych/Neuro
03/02/98	Psych/Neuro	Psych/Neuro	Psych/Neuro	Psych/Neuro	Psych/Neuro
03/09/98	Psych/Neuro	Psych/Neuro	Psych/Neuro	Psych/Neuro	Hum Sexuality
03/16/98	Hum Sexuality	Hum Sexualtiy	ACS	Free day	Exam 6

Note: ACS = Advanced Clinical Skills; CPC = Clinicicopathologic Conference; GI = Gastrointestinal Tract; Heart = Heart and Circulation; ID = Infectiuous Diseases; Immuno = Immunology; Neuro = Neurology and Neuropathology; PH I–IV = Pharmacology tutorial; Pysch = Psychiatry; Reprod = Reproduction; Rheum = Rheumatology.

of related or overlapping content usually are placed contiguous to one another and covered on the same examination. For example, Heart and Circulation follows Renal, with hypertension covered at the end of Renal and the beginning of Heart and Circulation. Gastrointestinal Tract and Liver are adjacent, as are the Endocrine, Reproduction, and Bone and Connective Tissue sections. Neurology, Psychiatry, and Human Sexuality are the final organ-based sections of year 2.

The last two days of the year are devoted to an orientation for the clinical rotations (formerly entitled Advanced Clinical Skills), which includes lectures such as "The Physician and the Pharmacy," "Prescription Writing," "Information Systems," and "The Electronic Patient Record," and a small-group hospital orientation led by fourth-year students.

The integration of courses varies by section but, overall, continues to increase as memories of the old curriculum fade and the new curriculum becomes better established. In the Microbiology and Infectious Diseases section and the Blood section, for example, pathology and Human Pathophysiology are virtually indistinguishable. Pharmacology, because of its focus on therapeutics, remains distinct from the other courses, but it is becoming more familiar to the focus groups and its content better integrated with other courses. The improved integration of the second-year curriculum is evident in the reduction of unintentional repetition, better coordination of content between the three core courses, and increased use of multidisciplinary symposia and case-based discussions.

The Future

It became apparent in recent years that a great disparity exists between the workloads in the first and second years, mostly because of the truncated nature of year 2. Further expansion of the second-year curriculum is impossible because of time constraints. After discussions with Dr. De Angelis and the coordinators of year 1 and year 2, it was decided that the Behavior component of the current second-year Psychiatry section could be integrated comfortably into the Neuroscience section of year 1. This move would decompress year 2 and add some clinically applicable material to year 1, both desirable goals. Psychiatry had previously been taught in year 1 but was moved into year 2 in the first iteration of the new curriculum. Since it was not feasible or desirable to add another quarter to year 2, the coordinators of year 1 and year 2 agreed that it would be better to move Behavior back to year 1 than to split the Microbiology and Infectious Diseases section by moving microbiology to year 1.

Beginning in the academic year 1998/99, fifty hours of the Behavior section was integrated into the first-year Neuroscience course. The year 2 Psychiatry section has retained the entire current pharmacology portion. Human Pathophysiology will focus on abnormal behaviors, with an emphasis on those that are relevant to therapeutics. With the rapid increase in our understanding of the biologic basis of abnormal behavior and of psychiatric therapy, it is likely that the Psychiatry section in year 2 will continue to grow and change.

One potential disadvantage of the current organ-system-based integration of year 2 is that while there has been great progress in vertical integration (integration between consecutive courses), there is little horizontal integration (integration between courses at the same level) and hence little emphasis on the interdependence of the organ systems. For example, the students learn about blood glucose control, islet cell pathology, and insulin therapy in the Endocrine section, but they learn about diabetic nephropathy in the Renal section and diabetic retinopathy in the Eye section. The excellent student makes the connections between systems; however, it is unfortunate that under the current time constraints the vertically integrated Human Pathophysiology, Pathology, and Pharmacology courses cannot cover the horizontal integration of organ systems. We are planning to use a portion of the additional time in year 2 for that purpose. The exact form of these new modules is undecided. We are considering topics such as diabetes, systemic lupus erythemetosis, and shock because of their multisystem manifestations.

The course directors are also discussing the development of a comprehensive, integrated final exam that will include material from the Human Pathophysiology, Pathology, and Pharmacology courses. Ideally, this exam would incorporate Clinical Skills. This would be accomplished by making part of the exam patient-based, by using either standardized patients or interactive computer programs. We envision the exam as requiring students to interview a patient and obtain a relevant history, accurately assess abnormal physical findings, interpret laboratory values and pathologic images, understand the relevant pathophysiology, and determine appropriate therapy. Such a multidisciplinary exam is an ambitious goal. This year we hope to administer, to volunteers, a pilot version of an integrated exam in Human Pathophysiology, Pathology, and Pharmacology. This exam will be constructed around patient scenarios. Involvement of standardized patients or interactive computer programs will require a great deal of time and planning in close collaboration with the Offices of Medical Education Services and Medical Informatics Education.

To use the added time in year 2, we plan to increase the number of lectures and small-group sessions that address the organ-specific topics of prevention and evidence-based medicine. To better integrate the year 1 and year 2 curricula, we have added lectures and small-group sessions on the epidemiology of specific diseases. This year there are lectures on the epidemiology of lung cancer and osteoarthritis. These lectures apply the basic principles taught in year 1 to specific disease processes and to clinical care. We plan to expand this series of lectures in the future.

One aim, not yet realized, is the integration of Clinical Skills with the core curriculum. This may require moving the beginning of Clinical Skills teaching, that is, history taking and the normal physical examination, into the first year. To do so would require a major alteration in the first year, which at this point is being considered.

Overall, the process of second-year curricular reform has been relatively pain free. Many people contributed to the success of the transition, particularly Dean Michael Johns and Vice Dean Catherine De Angelis, who provided unfailing support and enthusiasm. The Gang of Four/Five worked extraordinarily hard to conceptualize the changes and then to implement them. The directors of Pathology and Pharmacology provided input and guidance and ceded some autonomy. The focus-group leaders and members and the rest of the faculty entered enthusiastically into the new plan. Finally, the students provided invaluable input, especially during the first few years. We view the second-year curriculum as a living organism that requires constant nurturing for continued growth. The goal is to provide our students with the best possible preparation for the clinical curriculum and a foundation for lifelong learning.

5

Physician and Society

Leon Gordis, M.D., and Henry M. Seidel, M.D.

There is a growing recognition of the need to broaden the substance of medical education. Although most graduating medical students are well trained in bench laboratory sciences, diagnosis, and treatment, many have only limited knowledge of important aspects of physician-patient communication and are unaware of the influence of cultural factors in communication and in medical practice in general. Many new physicians lack knowledge of the basic biomedical ethics involved in the clinical dilemmas they will ultimately face. They also lack sufficient understanding of the social and economic aspects of health care, an understanding that is essential if they are to deal successfully with the rapidly changing structure and financing of health care in the United States.

The shift to managed care has led to a progressive depersonalization of the physician-patient relationship and increasing control of that relationship by peripherally involved nonphysicians whose bottom line is profit. The adequacy of physicians' compensation is often linked to an imposed directive to spend less time with each patient. Physicians also face ethical challenges when they confront health plan restrictions on the numbers and types of tests they may order and the numbers and types of specialist referrals they may make. For many physicians, these constraints are their first exposures to issues that have not been addressed in their medical education. They lack the foundation of knowledge and experience that would foster a determination to confront external pressures and enhance their relationships with their patients.

Finally, physicians are so pressured that many do not recognize that much of life's richness is to be gained from an appreciation of the arts. The pleasure of nontechnical and nonprofessional reading, including fiction and drama, is often lost on the new physician, whose only recollection of such reading may be from a required high school or college course in the distant past.

Institutional History

In 1991, the Johns Hopkins University School of Medicine decided to develop a course to address these issues as part of its overall curricular revision. The need for such a course had been suggested by the Brieger committee, which Dean Richard Ross had appointed in 1986 to examine the whole curriculum and to consider possible directions for change. The course that ultimately emerged, called Physician and Society (PAS), involved all four years of a student's medical school experience. The revision of the whole curriculum, including this course, was greatly facilitated by a generous grant from the Robert Wood Johnson Foundation. It is important to note that the decision to develop such a course was made before the school applied for the grant and that Dean Michael Johns was committed to the course regardless of the outcome of the grant application. Clearly, however, the grant funds greatly facilitated the development of PAS and made certain features possible that could not have been implemented in the absence of funding.

Planning Process and Chronology

The revised curriculum was planned one year at a time, beginning with the class that entered in September 1992. Thus, although PAS was a four-year course, the initial planning focused on the first year. The only directives given the course planners were that the new PAS course should incorporate two previously existing independent courses, History of Medicine and Medical Ethics, and should occupy two hours per week in the first-year curriculum.

The PAS planning committee was drawn from many departments of the school of medicine, in both clinical medicine and basic sciences. Initially, we selected the committee members on the basis of our personal acquaintance with them and our familiarity with their broad interests. The course director presented his plans to a meeting of the Advisory Board of the Medical Faculty, composed of all the department directors, and to a general meeting of the school of medicine faculty. At the latter meeting, interested faculty were invited to contact the course director, and several from various departments responded. Now that PAS is well known in the school of medicine and in other divisions of the university, additional faculty have come forward and taken on important roles in the course.

The objectives of PAS were to strengthen the physician-patient relationship and enhance the effectiveness of physician-patient communication. To achieve these objectives, the planning committee articulated a series of specific goals:

A. Transmit knowledge of ethical theory, biomedical ethics, and ethical analysis so that students will
   1. understand their ethical obligations to their patients, their families and friends, their colleagues, their communities, and society as a whole;
   2. appreciate the ethical dilemmas encountered in patient care and research and those posed by the structure of the health care system; and
   3. be able to apply ethical analysis to specific clinical cases that pose ethical problems.
B. Teach the history of medicine so that students will
   1. understand the historical evolution of the physician's role, the doctor-patient relationship, and the historical evolution of the relation between the physician and society; and
   2. appreciate the new ethical issues and challenges that have emerged as clinical medicine and medical research evolve.
C. Teach basic knowledge of cultural anthropology, sociology, law, and health economics so that students will
   1. understand the complexity of interaction among biobehavioral, socioeconomic, and cultural influences on the health of individuals and societies;
   2. understand how issues of cultural background, ethnic background, and gender must be taken into account in the provision of effective health care; and
   3. be aware of both subtle and overt manifestations of gender and racial bias.
D. Teach the basic principles of disease prevention so that students will
   1. understand that both prevention and treatment are integral parts of the physician's role and responsibility;
   2. appreciate the population concepts underlying both primary and secondary prevention and treatment of disease; and
   3. recognize the opportunities for prevention of occupationally and environmentally induced disease through both policy and regulation and through changes in individual life style.
E. Transmit knowledge of the global dimensions of health and disease so that students will
   1. appreciate the contrasting patterns of disease in developed and developing countries and the changes taking place;
   2. appreciate the different needs for preventive and therapeutic services in different societies; and

3. understand the effects of the interrelationships among different countries on the problems of health and disease worldwide.
F. Introduce students to the varied and changing societal perceptions of health and disease as expressed in various forms, such as drama, the visual arts, and scholarly writings, so that students will
   1. understand how society perceives both illness and physicians as well as other health care providers;
   2. appreciate the ways in which knowledge of the arts can enrich their professional lives as physicians; and
   3. understand that knowledge of the arts can be a broadly enriching experience, above and beyond the professional component of their lives.
G. Stimulate students to become lifelong learners through thinking, writing, analyzing, problem solving, and engaging in discussions so that they will
   1. develop a breadth of understanding of medicine and science, including the use of scientific methods;
   2. understand the relationship of scientific advances to the clinical practice of medicine;
   3. develop insight into the subjective realms of their patients' experiences with illness, uncertainty, dependency, and fear; and
   4. develop a respect for others and appropriate humility in their professional roles.

Two years later, the PAS faculty held a retreat to reexamine the goals, objectives, and functioning of the course and decided to retain the goals in their original form.

Structure and Configuration of the Course

The Physician and Society course meets for a two-hour session once a week in the first year and in the first three quarters of the second year, and twice a month in the third and fourth years. It includes frequent small-group interactions, which provide opportunities for discussion of the topics raised in class and give students a chance to learn about their classmates and to appreciate their diverse backgrounds and values. The goal is not to achieve *tolerance* in the sense of "putting up" with people thought to be of lesser stature or value. Rather, it is to help students learn to understand and respect their peers, sometimes coming to agree with them and adopting their point of view as their own, sometimes agreeing to disagree but respecting the positions expressed. This goal is emphasized in recognition of the fact that, throughout their lives, these future physicians will encounter varied values and attitudes in both their professional colleagues and their patients.

Overall, PAS is designed to address all of the goals of the course as listed above. The four years are viewed as a continuum in two ways. First, each year new material and topics are introduced that have not been presented before. Second, concepts and topics introduced in the previous year or years are addressed again in a different form and in a reinforcing fashion. Thus, the course embraces a series of themes that run through the four years, with variations.

The directors of the overall four-year course plan and implement the content of the second year in detail each year. The first, third, and fourth years have separate monitors who work in conjunction with the directors. The early years for any new course are clearly a period of trial and error: changes are made each year that reflect the prior year's experience and the philosophy of the current course director. In the PAS course, student input and evaluations have been critical in leading the directors to make major modifications. Moreover, by its nature a course such as this changes significantly from year to year in response to emerging current issues, which are incorporated into the content. In the sections below, we present the content for each year of PAS as taught in 1995/96; we have not included the various iterations that led to the schedule in that year.

Course Schedule in the First Year of PAS

The first-year PAS course meets weekly on Wednesdays from 11 A.M. to 1 P.M. It introduces students to major issues in medical ethics, the history of medicine, medical economics, culture and medicine, and physician-patient communication (table 5.1). Each session consists of a relatively brief lecture for the entire class followed by small-group discussions. The class includes students with a range of undergraduate majors from science to English and the arts. Many have minimal if any experience in a clinical setting. Therefore, the first year of medical school may be viewed as a fifth year of college, or at least as a transition from college to medical school. The PAS curriculum needs to adapt to the new students' study habits and classroom behaviors, with a view to fostering desirable changes.

Over the years, the PAS course has been planned with occasional blank sessions called "Hot Topics," which provide time for the study of issues that attract significant attention in the media or elsewhere. During the last presidential campaign, for example, a Hot Topic session was devoted to the major candidates' election platforms in regard to health. The blank sessions also allow the class to capitalize on visits to Johns Hopkins by distinguished guests.

Table 5.1   Schedule for Year 1 of Physician and Society

September 3	Overview of Four-Year Physician and Society Course

Dean's Introduction to Physician and Society

September 11	Introduction to Year 1

History of Medicine

September 18	Enduring Aspects
September 25	Hippocrates and the Hx of Medical Oaths
October 2	A Model of Its Kind: The History of Medicine at Johns Hopkins
	History of Women in American Medicine
October 9	Alternative and Complementary Medicine
October 23	History paper due

Ethics

October 23	Introduction to Medical Ethics
October 30	Ethical Theory
November 6	Autonomy and Beneficence
November 13	Confidentiality
November 20	Informed Consent
November 27	Holiday
December 4	Truth Telling
December 11	Conflicts of Interest
December 18	Essay exam due
December 18	HOT TOPIC SESSION
December 21	Winter break

Health Economics

January 8	Access to Care
January 15	Physician Reimbursement
January 22	Outcomes Research
January 29	Health Policy and Health Economics
February 5	Law and Medicine: Medical Malpractice and Informed Consent
February 12	Law and Medicine: Life, Death, Privacy, and the Law
February 19	Law and Medicine: Reproductive Rights and the Law
February 26	Introduction to Patient-Physician Communication: Recognition of Depression during Medical Visits
March 5	Communication of Medicine: Persuasive Communication and Smoking Cessation, Part 1
March 12	Communication of Medicine: Persuasive Communication and Smoking Cessation, Part 2
March 12	Essay exam due
March 19	Spring break

(*continued*)

Table 5.1   *(continued)*

Culture and Medicine

March 26	Spirituality and Medicine, Part 1: Panel Discussion
April 2	Spirituality and Medicine, Part 2: Small Groups
April 9	Issues in Racism, Part 1: Panel Discussion
April 16	Issues in Racism, Part 2: Small Groups
April 23	Minority Youth
April 30	Community project summary due

Advocacy and Activism

May 7	Legislative Lobbying
May 14	Public Health Policy
May 21	Public Health Policy
May 28	Take-home final exam due
June 4	Career Options

Course Schedule in the Second Year of PAS

In the Johns Hopkins medical school, clinical rotations begin in the final quarter of the second year. As a result, the second-year PAS schedule runs only through March, the end of preclinical course work in that year.

The second year of PAS, which is planned as a prelude to the clinical work, builds on the topics and material presented in the first year. A major unit is physician-patient communication. It includes two sessions in which students practice interviewing standardized patients, who exhibit various attitudes and emotions. Other sessions are devoted to the experience of minorities, women, and gays and lesbians as they confront the health care system. The second year also addresses issues related to personal boundaries, for example, those between private and professional life.

In 1995, "selectives" were introduced into the second year of PAS. These five-week minicourses, offered at the beginning of the year, were introduced at the suggestion of students who had finished the second year and met with the course directors to offer their evaluations. Ten selectives are offered in the first five weeks; they are repeated in the second five weeks. Before the first round, students rank their choices in order of descending interest, and as many students as possible are assigned to their top choice. The same procedure is followed in the second round. The selectives are popular with students. Those offered in 1996/97 included

—Ethical and Social Issues at the Beginning of Life
—Topics in Health Policy
—Medicine as Science and Medicine as Art: The Changing Role of Medicine in Twentieth-Century American Society
—Social Histories of the Patient
—Ethical and Social Issues in Clinical Genetics
—Disease: Historical Perspectives
—Unhealthy Jobs, Unhealthy Places: Occupational and Environmental Medicine
—Ethical and Social Issues at the End of Life
—The Laboratory and Medicine
—Medical Decision Making

A class of 120 divided into ten sections affords an excellent size for group discussion. The discussion group leaders are enthusiastic and generally are pleased by the fact that most students in their groups are self-selected. The selective approach also lends itself to flexibility in teaching methods. For example, students in the Occupational Medicine selective take field trips to industrial settings to examine occupational health problems firsthand. For many, this is their first exposure to industry. The logistics of arranging this type of experience are complex but workable for a group of twelve students (table 5.2).

Course Schedule in the Third and Fourth Years of PAS

Early in the planning of the third and fourth years of PAS, we decided to mix third- and fourth-year students in the same discussion groups. The rationale was twofold. First, we believed that third-year students could learn much from fourth-year students. Although the two groups mingle in some clinical rotations, this does not occur regularly, and the curriculum offers no organized activity that assures extended contact between third- and fourth-year students. Second, finding a sufficient number of appropriate group leaders for a course of this kind was a continual challenge. Moreover, many fourth-year students would miss sessions while traveling to internship interviews, and others would be enrolled in external electives off-campus. Anticipating this, it was reasonable to create larger groups.

PAS sessions in the third and fourth years are primarily small groups, although the classes meet as a whole from time to time. Some of the group discussions are devoted to readings of appropriate short stories. However, the main

Table 5.2   Schedule for Year 2 of Physician and Society

Selectives

September 10	Introduction to Selectives
September 17	Selective 1
September 24	Selective 1
October 1	Selective 1
October 8	Selective 1
October 15	Selective 1
October 22	Selective 2
October 29	Selective 2
November 5	Selective 2
November 12	Selective 2
November 19	Selective 2

Law and Medicine

November 26	Law and Medicine, Part 1
December 3	Law and Medicine, Part 2

Ethics

December 10	Ethics, Part 1
December 17	Ethics, Part 2

Patient-Physician Communication

January 7	Patients Affected by Substance Abuse or Dependence
January 14	Women in Medicine
January 21	Standardized Patients, Part 1
January 28	Standardized Patients, Part 2
February 4	Medical Student/Physician and the Lesbian, Gay, or Bisexual Person
February 11	Minorities

Boundaries in Medical Professionalism

February 18	Boundary Issues in Medicine
February 25	When Doctors Are Patients
March 4	Boundary Issues in Research
March 11	Conflicts of Interest and the Pharmaceutical Industry

focus is capitalizing on the clinical experiences of the students and using the experiences they have found particularly significant—in either positive or negative ways—as the basis for group discussions (table 5.3).

Freeing third- and fourth-year students from their clinical rotations was possible only with the strong support of the dean of the school of medicine. Dean

Table 5.3   Schedule for Years 3 and 4 of Physician and Society

September 19	Orientation
	Introductory Seminar[a]
October 3	Seminar: Literature ("The Bet," by Anton Chekhov)
October 17	Seminar: Literature ("The Insane," by William Carlos Williams)
November 7	Seminar: Literature ("Jean Beicke," by William Carlos Williams)
November 21	Seminar: Student Clerkship Experiences
December 5	Seminar: Student Clerkship Experiences
December 19	Panel Presentation: Johns Hopkins Medicine Fifty Years Ago
January 2	Seminar: Medical Ethical Dilemmas (Issues Involving Adolescents, Issues in Transplantations)
January 16	Seminar: Medical Ethical Dilemmas (Issues Involving Colleagues, Issues Involving Managed Care)
February 6	Seminar: Faith, Religion, and Medicine
March 6	Seminar: Student Clerkship Experiences
April 3	Seminar: Student Clerkship Experiences
April 17	Panel Presentation: Women Physicians at Johns Hopkins

[a]All seminars meet in small groups of fifteen students or fewer.

Johns sent a letter informing all department chairs and clerkship directors at the Johns Hopkins Hospital and affiliated hospitals that students would be absent from their clinical rotations twice a month on Thursdays from 8 to 10 A.M. The letter stated that PAS was not an elective but was required for promotion and graduation. We recognized the inconvenience for students of missing rotations, and it was for this reason that we scheduled only two PAS sessions per month for the clinical years. The hours of 8 to 10 A.M. were chosen to reduce the amount of clinical time lost in travel.

Coffee and bagels are served at 7:30 A.M., before the group discussions. While this was initiated as a gracious compensation for the early hour, it brought unanticipated benefits. It is one of the few times that third- or fourth-year students see their classmates as a group after completing their preclinical coursework, and it has proved to be a high point of the PAS experience. It gives students an opportunity to reinforce their bonding as a class. They are also able to chat informally with the faculty group leaders before beginning the group sessions.

The Grading System

To compete successfully for students' attention, PAS had to be a required course, one that students must pass to be promoted to the next year and to graduate. With 120 students in each class, there was no easy grading system. But pass/fail evaluations were not a realistic option as long as other courses gave letter grades; even the most motivated and enthusiastic students might neglect a pass/fail course in the effort to keep up with other required courses.

The substance of the coursework in PAS does not lend itself to multiple-choice tests or other quantitative assessments. We therefore rely on papers and projects for evaluation. Ideally, all 120 papers turned in for a particular assignment would be graded by one individual. However, as this is not possible, each small-group leader is asked to grade the students in his or her group. This approach offers the advantage of assessment by a faculty member who knows those students. However, students are appropriately concerned about equity, particularly in the absence of clear quantitative measures. They can be resentful when one group leader seems to be a tougher grader than another. This issue is not yet resolved.

A related issue is our decision to include the quality of student participation in group discussions as an element in the course grade. After much faculty discussion of the fairness of such a policy, a student commented that it was quite appropriate to grade on participation since physicians are expected to be able to communicate effectively with their physician colleagues and with other health care providers. However, the issue of subjectivity and variability among group leaders must always be kept in mind.

Evaluating the Course

In a new course, particularly one that differs so much from the traditional preclinical and clinical experiences, course evaluation is essential. Still, when many small-group discussions take place simultaneously, it is not possible for one person to learn enough about each group to make a valid assessment and comparison. Thus, frequent student evaluations are needed. During the first year PAS was offered, students submitted evaluations weekly, following each session. This frequency proved too high, as there was insufficient time to assimilate all the data generated. Very infrequent evaluations are problematic because of the potential for limited recall. It worked best to have students assess the course at the end of each unit. For example, the student evaluations submitted at the end of each selective in the second year have been invaluable to the planning committee in making appropriate changes and planning for the coming year.

Many of the faculty also serve as excellent evaluators. PAS faculty meetings are held several times a year to try to keep the simultaneous discussion groups on the same wavelength. At these meetings, faculty talk about what has worked and what has not worked, and make suggestions for appropriate changes.

Clearly, the ideal course evaluation would be based on a long-term outcome measure: does the course influence students' performance as physicians years later? Outcome evaluation, however, is extremely difficult. There are too many intervening variables, and the greater the time interval between the course and the performance assessment, the less relevant the data. Furthermore, for this course the outcome data tend to be qualitative—that is, based on anecdotal information obtained from clinical preceptors or other faculty—and they are not yet systematically collected. In practical terms, it is the immediate ongoing evaluations that are essential to improving the course.

Unanticipated Benefits

Although the goals of PAS were clearly articulated at the beginning of the course, benefits not originally expected have emerged. The small groups serve as forums in which students discuss many latent anxieties and concerns: "Do I belong in medical school?" "How can I balance my profession and my obligations to my family?" "I feel very lonely and isolated as a medical student—all my old friends are gone." "I am frightened of contracting a serious illness from my patients." Classmates serve as an excellent support network for students raising such issues in this setting. In addition, many quasi-advisor relationships have developed between students and small-group leaders, which help students address these and broader career issues. The course provides a setting in which positive mentor relationships develop.

PAS has also served as a binding force for faculty from various departments and disciplines, many of whom did not know each other outside the framework of this course. In particular, it has provided cohesiveness and visibility to a group of faculty interested in issues of ethics and physician communication. This group has become a valuable institutionwide resource.

Challenges

Recruiting PAS faculty is a continual challenge. Attrition is inevitable, even among the most motivated faculty, as competing obligations, illness, or other obstacles keep them from making the considerable time commitment required. A few persons simply lose enthusiasm after teaching the course for several years.

As a result it becomes necessary each year to identify new faculty. These individuals must have interests consistent with the content of PAS, be motivated to participate, and be appropriate as potential group leaders. Although retired and semiretired faculty are an excellent pool of talent and experience from which to recruit group leaders, it is important that a significant number be relatively young so that students can relate to them easily and perceive them as relevant role models. We have made every effort to recruit faculty from both the clinical (medical and surgical) and basic science departments.

Another challenge is the need for continuous revisions in course content, which are essential if the course is to maintain its vitality. These revisions must respect the variability of student interests and keep pace with societal changes. A collection of readings is developed for each year and revised annually. The absence of a specific text makes some students uncomfortable and leads them to conclude that the course is "soft" despite the many required readings. For this reason, we distribute as many of the readings as possible at the beginning of the year.

The approach to sensitive issues such as abortion remains problematic for a student body that is diverse ethnically, religiously, politically, and in other ways. To maintain its relevance, PAS must confront difficult, contentious issues. Constructive discussion and amicable disputation of such issues requires great skill and a feeling of comfort on the part of the group leader.

To succeed, a course like PAS needs strong support from the dean and the vice dean for academic affairs and faculty. That support can counter the resistance of some faculty to yielding part of their teaching time to the course and the perception of others that space in the curriculum should not be devoted to such topics. While faculty resistance has not been a significant problem at Johns Hopkins, the commitment to the course from the start by the administrative leaders of the medical school and by the university president, Dr. William Richardson, was invaluable.

The PAS course is expensive. It makes extensive demands on the time of faculty and support staff: more than sixty faculty members from the school of medicine and the school of public health are involved each year. The university's limited resources allow for assuming only a minimal portion of PAS faculty salaries, and a faculty member's total salary does not increase as a result of participation. Clearly, the PAS faculty are highly dedicated, but their commitment is hard to maintain in an era of intense pressures on faculty to generate financial support of their salaries.

The first years of PAS were funded partly by a grant from the Robert Wood Johnson Foundation. With the end of the grant, the school of medicine faced the challenge of supporting the course by dedicating funds from its own budget. This has worked so far, but institutional budgets generally are formulated one year at a time. A course such as PAS requires a multiple-year commitment for planning and development, and to permit faculty to plan their involvement over a prolonged time.

The course directors and monitors play a major role. Ideally, the position of course director should be a 75 to 100 percent time commitment, although financial limitations make such an arrangement impractical. The director's role is not purely administrative: it involves developing the curriculum, meeting with students outside class, developing training sessions for faculty, and exploring comparable offerings at other institutions.

Another major challenge for the course director is to maintain the excitement felt by the faculty during the early years of the course. A sense of sameness sets in despite changes from year to year, and creative approaches are essential to maintain faculty enthusiasm.

PAS is a large undertaking. It is the only course in the school of medicine that simultaneously includes all 480 medical students spanning the four years of medical school. Maintaining continuity in planning over the four years is a critical and insistent challenge. To that end, we have taken one major step by designating a senior PAS faculty member as director of the ethics portion of the course for all four years. This individual makes sure that the four-year ethics content constitutes a logical continuum.

Another continuing challenge is assuring at least a minimum of uniformity among the seminar groups without stifling the digressions that may develop in any lively discussion. We have scheduled instructors' meetings in the evenings to address this issue. The meetings seem to be of value, but we are not yet content with the result.

The administrative responsibilities associated with this course are extensive. For example, the mundane task of obtaining rooms for all of the discussion groups is a significant problem. The scheduling of classes and meetings, the distribution of course materials to faculty and students, and the collection and logging-in of student assignments all are unusually time-consuming in a course this size.

Ideally, PAS should be integrated as much as possible with the rest of the curriculum. For example, when students learn genetics in a laboratory course, PAS might address the ethical issues of genetic screening. When students study developmental biology, PAS might cover the problems of caring for a child with a congenital malformation, perhaps also including the costs to society and the ethical dilemmas that may arise. However, the course cannot be entirely dependent on integration. It must maintain its particular content and identity.

A final challenge for PAS is the contrast between students' experiences in the classroom and in clinical settings. When students begin their clinical rotations, they often encounter house officers working under great pressure who tell them to de-emphasize physician-patient communication and to work as quickly as possible. Thus, the students confront a dilemma between respect for what they learn in PAS and the pragmatic impact of some of the role models they meet. Ultimately, PAS will need to involve house staff and perhaps attending physicians if the content of the preclinical years is to be carried over and reinforced in the students' clinical experiences and subsequent professional careers.

Conclusions

If one views the task of medical education from the perspective of a physician educated in the Flexnerian (traditional) mode, there is a compelling need for a course like Physician and Society. There were problems in medical education in Flexner's day—the early years of this century—and there are problems now. Education at the bedside too easily becomes a kind of "show and tell" in the hands of inadequate teachers (who may be excellent physicians) and harassed house officers. Clinical settings in an academic institution rarely resemble these in the outside world. And the selection process by which medical students are anointed has yet to come to grips with the subjective qualities that society seeks in the physician. Most students arrive at medical school practiced in the art of taking exams; once there they find too little opportunity to practice the art of medicine.

No wonder there is pressure to modify the traditional approach. To fill the perceived gap in the medical educational process is a daunting challenge, however. Society wants change but is not particularly willing to pay for it, and the medical profession is caught up in the stubborn defense of its territory and privileges. Physicians now face challenges related not only to the substance of physicianhood but to the territory and economic base of the profession.

It was in this context that the PAS directors pursued the development of the course, borrowing to some extent from similar efforts elsewhere. There is no question that foundation support was enabling, but the primary impetus and essential long-term commitment came from Deans Ross and Johns. The students themselves have been enormously helpful, and a cadre of interested faculty members has served as a necessary if not sufficient resource. Not all students respond positively to our effort, but most do. Many have given careful constructive criticism over the years. It is from these sources that the directors have found support in an environment that is still devoted—and rightly so—to the Flexnerian concept. We say rightly because there is nothing in Flexner that contradicts the aims of PAS. The two are complementary and, in the view of the directors, both essential in providing an environment where our students can realize their inherent potential.

We should not overstate the probable value of this course. No satisfactory outcome study exists. If, however, the environment of medical school is enhanced by PAS and if students feel that it enriches the experience of growing and developing as a physician, we can assert the value of the course and feel confirmed in the intention to continue.

The values taught in the Physician and Society course run the risk of being mere window dressing until students find positive reinforcement in the behavior and attitudes of the medical faculty and the profession as a whole. The contribution of the course ultimately will be small if we do not renew our efforts to understand what makes both competency and compassion possible in a physician. All of us as physicians must seek to imbue every relationship with a patient with a sense of complete understanding of that person's needs. The needs of the patient must inform our effort in every regard. There will be no substantial progress until this is habitual in what we do, and until there is societal recognition of the imperative to support this level of effort.

6

Medical Informatics, Educational Technology, and the New Curriculum

Harold P. Lehmann, M.D., Ph.D.

Information management in general, and computer use in particular, emerged as important medical education goals in the early 1980s (DeBliek, Friedman, and Purcell 1983). Medical schools have used a wide range of strategies in implementing these goals, with varying degrees of success (AAMC 1992). At Johns Hopkins, the William H. Welch Medical Library assumed a leadership role in bringing the scholarly use of electronic resources into the medical environment (Matheson and Cooper 1982), but despite some efforts in the mid-1980s, the medical school curriculum was relatively unaffected. The strategy we chose at Johns Hopkins was to build on the changes planned through the Robert Wood Johnson Foundation (RWJF) external grant that funded the medical school's general curricular reform. In the original grant proposal to the RWJF in 1989, we stated four computer-related principles: (1) computer software can help students acquire the knowledge they need for clinical decision making; (2) a collaborative, networked computer environment is essential for modeling the multidisciplinary clinical activities in which students will later take part; (3) a medical informatics curriculum can help to prepare students for the clinical world; and (4) researching new informatics methods and investigating the effectiveness of informatics activities in medical education are integral components of even routine use of computers in the curriculum.

Informatics is the use of the basic and applied sciences in dealing with the management of information and the support of decision making in medicine. In the grant application we suggested that medical informatics would have an impact on the following objectives of the schoolwide curricular reform project: computerizing learning and teaching; rewarding faculty for teaching; expanding the use of case-based, small-group learning sessions; integrating the basic sciences and clinical experiences; expanding ambulatory experiences; and incorporating social issues into the study of medicine.

The computer-and-informatics effort comprised two parts: educational technology, to support the curriculum, and medical informatics, to extend the curriculum. This chapter reviews the process for accomplishing these goals and evaluates its success so far.

Administrative Strategy

Instituting change in a medical school curriculum, even noninvasively, requires the concerted efforts of a number of administrative players. Our changes required cooperative action within the larger informatics context at Johns Hopkins. The main players in our story are the Division of Biomedical Information Sciences, the Welch Medical Library, and the Office of Medical Informatics Education (OMIE). Figure 6.1 shows the administrative structure pertinent to computers and informatics in 1992 and 1996.

The Division of Biomedical Information Sciences

Nina Matheson, Welch Medical Library director from 1984 to 1993, brought the library into the forefront by defining the relationship between the medical library and the scholarly activities associated with the academic medical center (Matheson and Cooper 1982). Following her retirement in 1993, the school of medicine took advantage of the opportunity to rethink that relationship and the possible mechanisms for providing campuswide computing support. The Division of Biomedical Information Sciences was created, and David T. Kingsbury, Ph.D., was appointed its director. He was also appointed director of the Welch Medical Library and, subsequently, associate dean for information sciences and chief information officer of the university.[1]

The Division of Biomedical Information Sciences, comprising both academic and service units, was responsible for providing non-patient-record information services for the Johns Hopkins Medical Institutions (JHMI). The division's role was to advance science and health through information management. This role was carried out by the division's four organizational entities: the Welch Medical Library, the Laboratory for Applied Bioinformatics, the JHMI Network and Telecommunications Service, and OMIE.

The library provided print and electronic resources, computing facilities for educational and general use, Internet access, and a wide array of courses; its role

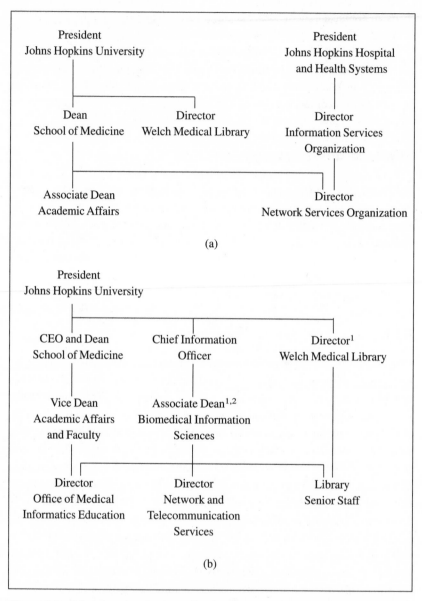

Figure 6.1 Administrative Structure Reporting pertinent to medical informatics in 1992 (a) and 1996 (b). [1] The director of the Welch Medical Library and the associate dean of biomedical information sciences are the same person. [2] This position is also the directorship of the Division of Biomedical Information Sciences.

is discussed more fully in the next section. The Laboratory for Applied Bioinformatics provided innovative information services for the biomedical community as a whole. The Network and Telecommunications Service was responsible for the general networking and computational infrastructure for all members of the JHMI. OMIE is discussed later in this chapter. In 1996, the Johns Hopkins Hospital's Information Services Organization was subsumed under the Johns Hopkins Medicine Center for Information Services; as a result, the academic and clinical groups developed a closer working relationship and a growing appreciation of one another's needs and technical solutions.

An early project of the Division of Biomedical Information Sciences was the creation of a campuswide information system called InfoNet (http://infonet.welch.jhu.edu). Built on the World Wide Web, InfoNet represented the institution's commitment to the electronic delivery of information, including educational content. InfoNet not only provided access to the World Wide Web but also offered educational programs and disseminated technology within the university.

The Welch Medical Library

The William H. Welch Medical Library (http://www.welch.jhu.edu), founded in 1929, serves the schools of medicine, public health, and nursing; the Johns Hopkins Hospital; and the Kennedy Krieger Institute. Its mission is to provide the JHMI and affiliates with information services that advance research, teaching, and patient care. The library provides services designed to help JHMI clients locate, select, and use knowledge resources anywhere in the world, regardless of the medium (paper, computer, or other). Particular emphasis is placed on access to electronic information. The library staff monitor the information needs of the medical community and develop products and services designed to meet those needs.

The Welch Medical Library operates an active education program covering instruction and research experiences at many educational levels. A wide variety of courses is provided in areas such as scientific writing; computer, Internet, and network skills; access to electronic information resources; and data analysis and presentation (Brandt and Campbell 1995; Stephens and Campbell 1995).

The library administers the Information Resource Center (IRC), the primary computer resource for medical students. During the implementation period under the RWJF grant, the complement grew to some forty computers, including Macintoshes and PCs. From the IRC, students have access not only to programs on the desktop machines but to E-mail and the World Wide Web. The computers are available twenty-four hours a day, seven days a week, although library staff are available only part of the time (they work day and evening hours on week-days and part of the day on weekends). Also in the course of this effort, four Macintosh computers were made available in the small-group teaching rooms of the Preclinical Teaching Building. This has made it possible for the computers to be used in teaching, and the larger space affords a greater opportunity for groups of students to learn together during unscheduled time.

A more widely available service administered by the library is Internet access for students and faculty through the Welchlink computer. The number of accounts grew exponentially in the mid-1990s, from five hundred in 1993 to ten thousand in early 1996, and dial-in access was provided. The Internet education program has expanded in parallel; it now includes an introductory and an intermediate course, a course in basic World Wide Web material preparation, and an annual two-day Internet Fair. Since 1993, all medical students have been automatically assigned an Internet account and required to attend an orientation session.

Because of the library's efforts, electronic communication and access to information have become an integral part of the work life at the JHMI.

The Office of Medical Informatics Education

The Office of Medical Informatics Education (http://omie.med.jhmi.edu) was established in March 1992, funded in part by the RWJF grant and the dean's office. It was created as a component of the dean's Office of Academic Affairs and, in 1995, became part of the Division of Biomedical Information Sciences. OMIE's purpose is to coordinate the informatics education of medical students, including training in the use of educational technology. OMIE's activities are described in more detail throughout this chapter.

Operating Strategy

The operating strategy, technical plan, and process of software development and integration for educational technology and informatics were implemented primarily through OMIE. The goals of the operating strategy were, and still are, to (1) increase the perceived need for computers and for informatics systems and training; (2) match the delivery of services to the perceived need; (3) provide high-quality materials; and (4) integrate materials and skills with the curriculum.

To increase the perceived need, OMIE has evangelized the faculty on the importance of educational technology and medical informatics. In 1993, Dr. Catherine De Angelis created the Committee for Computers in the Curriculum to enhance communication among faculty, staff, and students. This committee was successful in defining and creating a new course, the Literature Searching Practicum, described later in this chapter. The committee identified the lack of computers, especially in the clinical years, as a major problem in instituting a medical informatics curriculum. After this initial effort, the committee's work for directing general informatics development was transferred to the existing Educational Policy Committee (EPC).

OMIE staff spoke at divisional and departmental meetings to promote the use of computers in the curriculum, the teaching of computer skills, and informatics issues in general. The staff sent supplemental mailings and made follow-up phone calls to course directors and other teaching faculty members. OMIE and the library often sent representatives to the EPC's monthly meetings to discuss the possible usefulness or relevance of educational technology and medical informatics in the curriculum and in the administration of courses.

The library collaborated with OMIE to publicize informatics issues via the quarterly newsletter *Welch Library Issues.* In September 1994, the library, the Department of Art as Applied to Medicine, the Department of Pathology Photography, and OMIE presented an "Info-Fair," where faculty, students, and staff could see or learn about the computer-related educational resources available on campus.

To gain allies outside the school of medicine, OMIE and the library began sending representatives to the university-wide Subcommittee on Electronic and Distance Education (http://www.jhu.edu/sede), which addresses issues ranging from long-distance charges for the transmission of video signals on telephone lines to the administration of an internal mini-grant program to foster electronic and distance education. OMIE and the library have also provided consulting services to the Department of Art as Applied to Medicine, the school of public health, the school of nursing, and the University Design and Publications Group.

To gain allies outside the JHMI altogether, OMIE served as the university's representative to the National Education Medical School Consortium (NEMSC), a group of fifteen medical schools committed to developing computer-based materials and to sharing them with one another.[2] (See A. R. Dwak et al. [1994] on the importance of consortium membership and codevelopment in furthering local educational technologies.) The medical school obtained high-quality software through the consortium, shared its own software creations, and benefited from critiques of its software by other schools. Another external link was with the National Library of Medicine. OMIE played a vital role in several phases of that library's cardiac embryology project, primarily by obtaining user evaluations and design feedback.

To provide high-quality materials and to integrate materials and skills into the curriculum, OMIE took on the task of software development. Although this tactic is expensive, it is justified on several counts. First, integrators of educational technology in medical schools are well acquainted with the "NIH" (Not Invented Here) syndrome: if a software package is not created at the medical school, faculty are reluctant to support it, let alone promote it. Thus, persuading faculty to use any software may entail development. Second, even purchased software needs to be customized, so development skills are necessary. Third, our commitment to materials of high technical quality necessitates the knowledge that only developers have. Nevertheless, OMIE continues to seek externally developed software, where possible.

OMIE's attempt to oppose the "NIH" syndrome on occasion—its refusal to support a few poorly specified pet projects for software development when comparable software was available for purchase—earned it a small number of detractors. But disagreements and critical faculty review have meant that, although Johns Hopkins students have fewer programs available than do students at some other schools, the programs are well used and thoughtfully integrated into the curriculum. For every program that is supported, a software handout is created, an in-class demonstration of the software is performed, and software availability is coordinated with the faculty's needs and the course schedule.

The Welch Medical Library and OMIE coordinate the delivery of educational computer services. The library is responsible for providing the computers and technical support (coordinating software availability requires 25 percent of a full-time technical-support employee), maintaining hardware and software, and supplying the staff who provide user assistance at the IRC.

Technical Plan

Our technical goal for computer-based education was to provide ubiquitous and continuous access to high-quality educational material through an education-enhancing interface. Ubiquity and continuity were necessary because the computer network is vital to the school's activities. High-quality computer-based educational material, evaluated through an academic review process, and high-quality software, evaluated by the standards set in the technical plan, were necessary to ensure that the interface would, in fact, enhance students' education.

Figure 6.2 shows the topology of this plan, which assumes a campuswide network backbone of sufficient bandwidth to supply educational software in the form of images, video, and Internet access. A server of educational software was also necessary, together with an adequate number of user sites. The IRC is a traditional computer lab. Although many of the programs are designed for a standalone configuration, we wanted a networked environment to allow Internet ac-

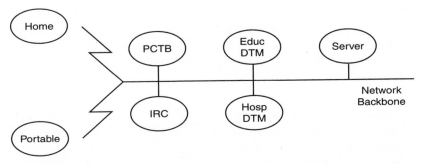

Figure 6.2   Ubiquitous and continuous access to educational material. DTM = desktop machine; IRC = the Information Resource Center; PCTB = Preclinical Teaching Building.

cess. The Preclinical Teaching Building is composed of lecture halls, teaching labs, and small-group learning spaces; we planned for computer technology to be used in these sites. We also planned for computer training and use during the clinical years, either at hospital-based desktop machines or at hospital-based education-oriented workstations. Finally, we assumed that students would need to access educational materials from home and from remote learning sites.

In 1994, Dr. Kingsbury made the Internet and the World Wide Web the central components of this systemwide technical plan. At that time, the available Web browsers were inferior to educational environments such as HyperCard® and ToolBook®. However, simple navigational functionality soon gave way to the complex capabilities that are needed today for effective, interactive educational software, and as a result we became committed to delivery of educational material to the Web wherever possible.

The Process of Introducing Educational Technology

We divided the process of introducing educational technology into the following units:

—development of faculty skills
—acquisition of content
—development of material
—integration of material
—delivery of material

For instance, to "find software" (acquisition of content) for the Microbiology course means doing the following: (1) finding out from faculty members what they need and demonstrating the possibilities of computers in teaching; (2) finding or creating software to satisfy those needs; (3) customizing purchased software for use at Johns Hopkins; (4) determining how the software should be used in the actual teaching of the course; and (5) supporting students in learning to use it.

To take the process through these phases requires a range of skills:

—political (evangelizing the faculty)
—instructional (matching instructional needs to the technology)
—programming (producing the software)
—editorial (ensuring accuracy of the educational content)
—technical support (getting the machinery to work)
—user support (helping the students)

In OMIE, the director was responsible for political and managerial efforts, the courseware design specialist was responsible for instructional aspects, and the software systems specialist was responsible for programming. A secretary rounded out the OMIE staff. Faculty experts performed the high-level editorial reviews. The Welch Library Information Technology Group was responsible for technical support, and the library reference staff provided user support. Of course, none of the lines drawn here are sharp; everyone used more than one of these skills. Appendix 6.1 gives a sense of the breakdown of work for 1995/96 along these dimensions. Below, we discuss these activities in detail.

The position of courseware design specialist proved to be the most difficult to defend to the administration, because the role was unfamiliar. (Faculty and staff members know what programmers are supposed to do because they often work with programmers in administration and research programming; this is not the case with courseware designers.) The original job description reads as follows:

> A senior designer is sought to manage and direct the efforts of the Courseware Development Laboratory [which later became OMIE] of the Johns Hopkins School of Medicine. The designer will work with the Director of Medical Informatics Education and interested faculty and students in developing courseware on the Macintosh platform for a novel curriculum in medical education. The position involves the performance of front-end analyses of courses and curricula, the design and development of appropriate human-computer interfaces, the management of product and project timelines, and the design and implementation of usability testing and summative analyses. Excellent skills in communication, teamwork, interface design, prototype development, and educationally principled design are required. Master's level or industry experience in educational technology are requisites.

Should possess the ability to:

a. Work closely with faculty in developing and designing computer-based interactive systems
b. Develop specifications and prototypes for computer-based instructional materials for medical students
c. Create storyboards and flow charts
d. Create instructional framework, concept development, and formative and summative evaluation plans
e. Research and recommend various hardware and software that will enhance the effectiveness of the Courseware Development Lab and the School of Medicine

Joan Freedman became OMIE's courseware design specialist. In addition to the tasks listed above, she took on major responsibilities in managing the various projects and organizing publicity. Day-to-day management of the software-loading schedule also consumed much time and effort.

Developing educational software in a medical school is challenging. Faculty time limitations and the press of the educational schedule work against the professional software development cycle of establishing specifications up front, designing features, and implementing the features in a recurrent cycle of faculty and end-user feedback (Lehmann 1995).

Medical Informatics

Our strategy for creating a coherent medical informatics curriculum across the four years was to (1) create a list of desired learning objectives for medical informatics; (2) determine where in the current curriculum those objectives were already satisfied; and (3) determine how to satisfy the other objectives. Part of the agenda for steps 1 and 2 was to educate current course directors about medical informatics. Much of this effort built on other OMIE activities, described earlier. Its results are reported below.

Assessment of Student Needs

An essential component of both informatics and educational technology is needs assessment. OMIE conducts annual surveys to assess students' informatics needs and has investigated the question of mandatory computer ownership by students. Each summer since 1993, the registrar has sent a one-page questionnaire to incoming students. The results are summarized in table 6.1. From these data, we concluded that (1) given the universal experience with word processing and other computer tools, students had a high degree of computer literacy;

Table 6.1 Results of Survey of Incoming Students on Informatics Needs

	1993	1994	1995	1996	1997
No. of respondents (% of class)	106 (88)	106 (88)	114 (95)	116 (97)	184[a]
Computers owned					
Macintoshes (% of owners)	32 (49)	34 (50)	32 (41)	35 (45)	38 (34)
PCs (DOS +Windows) (% of owners)	29 (45)	23 (34)	46 (59)	42 (55)	75 (66)
Total (% of respondents)	65 (61)	67 (76)	79 (69)	77 (66)	113 (61)
Modem owned (% of respondents)		22 (21)	43 (56)	56 (73)	94 (76)
Computer skills/experience (% of respondents)					
Word processing	96	100	97	97	96
Data analysis	73	74	72	64	73
Literature searching	n/a[b]	83	75	82	84
E-mail	66	67	84	90	92
World Wide Web	n/a	6	55	82	92

[a]Medical and graduate students combined.

[b]n/a = not asked.

138

(2) no more than 60 percent of students owned computers; and (3) because students were almost evenly split in the types of computers they owned, a single-platform (Mac or PC) policy would be wrong.

The dean's office has considered requiring computer ownership of all incoming students. We have postponed making a recommendation until the following are demonstrated: (1) a commitment by the faculty to put material online; (2) a commitment by the administration to support online interaction; and (3) a commitment by the administration to provide student user support. As of this writing, conditions 1 and 2 are met, but an adequate budget for user support is not yet available.

By 1996, the Johns Hopkins Hospital had installed a few desktop computers and planned to provide two computers to each ward in the following year. The students had forty-four computers available to them for learning, although none were in clinical areas. The Preclinical Teaching Building was fully networked in 1995, so that machines located in the teaching rooms, where students studied in groups for long periods, could be connected to each other and to the Internet.

Educational Technology Results

This section describes the curriculumwide results of the educational technology effort, including the LectureLinks curriculum repository; the results of two large development efforts, the Histology image database and the Respiratory Physiology tutorial; and the results of our curriculum support for each year of the curriculum.

One resource we created that spans the curriculum is the software database. In 1992, there were no electronic directories available to medical educators to advise them of available computer-based resources. (For instance, the Health Sciences Consortium database and the University of Michigan databases were not yet available. The latter was published in 1995 as *Software for the Health Sciences: An Interactive Resource,* with 740 entries [Learning Resource Center].) We needed a way of keeping track of our own experience with software evaluation, so we began a simply structured database to note all available computer programs. We used catalogs, conference proceedings, and other available material as sources for this database. By 1996, there were more than a thousand items in the database. We informed faculty members by mail about the availability of this resource. In the summer of 1994, we sent a packet to each first-year lecturer, containing entries from the software database that might be of interest. Apart from two who had already shown interest, no faculty members responded, despite follow-up phone calls. We discontinued work on the database.

Our collaboration with the Department of Art as Applied to Medicine has been more successful. Joan Freedman led a course there for several years on the design of computer-based educational materials. Students from that course have created images and animations for the medical students, either as part of the course or for their theses.

Our computer-use data in 1995 showed that more than 80 percent of students used the software we made available to them. The median session time in the IRC for educational software was ten minutes; the seventy-fifth percentile was at twenty minutes. Session times almost doubled in the small-group rooms, presumably because there was less pressure from other students waiting to use the computers.

LectureLinks

In the summer of 1995, Joan Freedman and a medical student named Melissa Marks-Sparrow (class of 1998) developed the idea that led to LectureLinks, our core World Wide Web curriculum repository (http://omie.med.jhmi.edu/LectureLinks/). In the course of the summer, Marks-Sparrow, with some help from her classmate Oletha Minto, collated the lectures of the first-year curriculum and found Web sites throughout the world that related to each lecture. From the outset, it was also a goal of LectureLinks to put local curriculum material, such as lecture notes, on-line. Figure 6.3 shows a representative page of this resource.

We quickly realized that LectureLinks would serve multiple uses and users. First, it would inspire students to start using the Web, a source of continuing, life-long learning. Second, it would provide a service to the students, not so much during a particular course but later, in the clinical years, when they would need to review the material, thus supporting "just-in-time" learning (learning at the time of need). Third, it would familiarize faculty members with topics taught by other faculty, serving as a curriculum database—a type of database that schools like the University of North Carolina at Chapel Hill (Mattern et al. 1992), the Medical College of Ohio (Nowacek, Miller, and Young 1995), and the University of Cincinnati College of Medicine (Stoner and Heider 1995) have spent much effort developing.

In the winter of 1995, the University Subcommittee on Electronic and Distance Education conducted a competition for small internal grants; LectureLinks was one of the projects awarded. (OMIE was not involved in the judging or selection process.) The purpose of the funding was to expand on the work of Marks-Sparrow and Minto by (1) organizing LectureLinks as a formal database; (2) hiring a medical artist to create course-related images to which John Hopkins would own the copyright; and (3) hiring a student to assist with the collection and re-

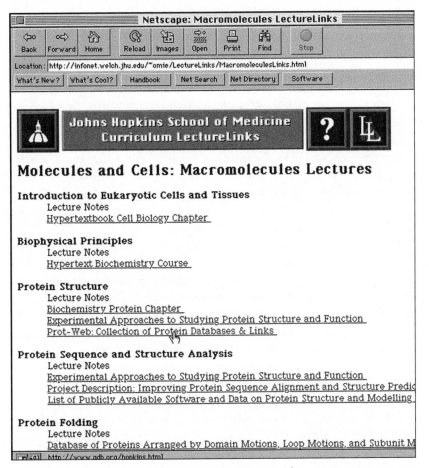

Figure 6.3   A LectureLinks Web page from 1996.

formatting of curricular material. We also convened a student advisory board of about twelve students during the four years of educational technology development to help make decisions on functionality, process, and Web site choices.

Simultaneously, we worked on bringing second-year course material, including teachers' lecture notes, into LectureLinks. Some course directors were cooperative, and we then faced a new set of difficulties: (1) the faculty used a variety of electronic methods for creating their notes; (2) copyrights were not cleared for the majority of notes; (3) some faculty thought that their notes were too sketchy or disorganized to appear on-line; and (4) some faculty were reluctant to put their notes on-line because they felt that the notes would then have to be of chapter-level (publishable) quality, entailing even more work. We gave faculty final say over the disposition of their lecture notes. We worked with those who agreed with our goals to surmount any technical difficulties.[3]

Histology Image Database

In 1993, Dr. Renee Dintzis asked OMIE to digitize the kodachrome teaching slides used in the Histology course. We determined the following needs for this project: (1) to make the slides available to more students at any one time; (2) to protect the slides against losses due to theft, damage, or misplacement; (3) to label all slides, directing students to their important contents; and (4) to use local slides because they were based on the microscopic slides that Johns Hopkins students used in their labs. The functional specifications for the program included browsing slides, searching for slides, and self-testing.

We created three versions of this resource while devising the final functionality: (1) a client-server database with only the slide image and little associated text; (2) a simplified version of the same information in FileMaker Pro®; and (3) a full-fledged application, called OverLayer, that can display slides and associated structures (integrated into a proprietary file format) and that includes self-testing functionality. OverLayer is a PICT image-browser application native to the Macintosh 680x0/PowerPC, which has the ability to display predefined QuickDraw regions of discontiguous areas or points within an image. Overlays may contain a text-string name and a short paragraph description. They define a region of an image by means of an outline or color wash, as used to be done with overheads and transparencies. In the case of the Histology Imagebase, they are applied to tissue components. An overlay may be identified by clicking on it directly or may be located by selecting its name from a scrolling list (fig. 6.4). In addition to displaying PICT images and layers, OverLayer contains a testing mode for identifying and/or locating a randomly selected layer within a randomly selected slide.

These three versions of the Kodachromes database were developed by programmer Martin Wachter. The content was developed by the course director, working with us and with student Laura Snyder (class of 1997) in particular, and also with Oletha Minto (class of 1998).

Our experience with OverLayer was presented at the Symposium on Computer Applications in Medical Care (Lehmann and Wachter 1995) and also at the Computers in Healthcare Education Symposium of the Health Sciences Library Consortium (Philadelphia, April 1995) (Lehmann 1995). The program has been shared with the NEMSC, as well. Students' enthusiasm for this program is indicated by their willingness to schedule computer time into the early hours of the morning because of high demand.

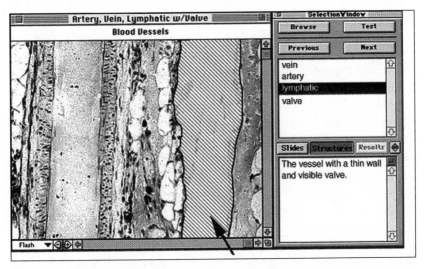

Figure 6.4   The Histology OverLayer application, with image window displaying a selected tissue structure.

Creating this image database involved three steps: (1) digitizing the slides; (2) postprocessing the slides; and (3) archiving the slides. Digitizing the slides required a slide scanner and appropriate software. Postprocessing involved touching up artifacts, brightening the images, and adding labels and other educational elements. Archiving involved putting the large amount of data generated into the appropriate format, e.g., for a CD-ROM or file server.

Labeling the slides involved (1) a faculty member to specify which structures should be labeled; (2) a student or interested faculty member to outline manually each structure in the slide (by using a commercially available graphics program such as Canvas®) and to attach the text label, description, and question and answer for each layer; (3) a faculty member to check the outlining and text; and (4) a programmer to integrate the slide, outline, and text into the OverLayer format.

Students are particularly fond of this program, not only because of its functionality but because of its close relationship to the content of the Histology course. Although most faculty members feared that use of computers would interfere with the learning of important skills, student scores in the microscope practicum of the Histology course have risen each year with the increasing use of this program by students. We are in the process of a formal evaluation of the impact of the program on students and faculty in the Histology laboratory course.

Our long-term plan is to move the image database to the World Wide Web to make it available in the clinical years and throughout the Johns Hopkins extended campus. We received funding from the National Library of Medicine through a Library Resources (G08) grant to reimplement this project in the Java language and to create a modest library of a thousand digitized, labeled images in domains beyond Histology (namely, Pathology and Gastroenterology). Dr. Dintzis also obtained funding through a provost's grant (similar to that for Lec-tureLinks) to expand the content of the image database and to make a formal eval-uation of the use of the program during lab time.

Finally, in creating the database content, we formulated functional or physi-ologic questions for each slide. This question bank—yoked to the images—serves as a self-teaching (and self-grading) resource. It has also been reimple-mented on the Web (http://omie.med.jhmi.edu/hist).

Respiratory Physiology Tutorial

Our other major development effort has been in physiology. The physiology de-partment has been a consistent early adopter of computer technology. Even be-fore the educational technology effort, the Cardiac Physiology section used a cardiac-dynamic simulator, developed by Drs. Dan Burkhoff and Lowell Maughan, as a laboratory required of all students.[4] The simulator subsequently was adapted by Dr. David Kass as a computer-based cardiac physiology labora-tory required of all students. This laboratory presents computer-simulation data generated as if in real time, so that students can manipulate the simulated heart much as investigators used to do to real isolated hearts. The involvement of the students with the discovery process and the fact that the simulation responds to both correct and incorrect choices has proved extremely valuable as a teaching tool. More recent efforts, under the leadership of Organ Systems course director Dr. William Guggino, have been to create a computer-based respiratory physi-ology curriculum and to use Internet services as effectively as possible for course administration.

For the Respiratory Physiology section, along with section leader Dr. Wilmot Ball, we began in 1992 to develop a tutorial computer program aimed at topics that Dr. Ball and students had identified over the years as particularly difficult to learn: the pressure-volume changes during normal breathing and the pressure-compliance relationships with open and closed glottis, among others. We ini-tially created a stand-alone version of the program, which is named Interactive Respiratory Physiology, with much content development by medical student Rachel McCormick (class of 1996). In its first year (1994), the tutorial was used by 80 percent of the students for twenty to forty minutes at a time, demonstrat-ing its use for primary learning. On an end-of-year questionnaire, 73 percent of the respondents confirmed the program's usefulness in learning.

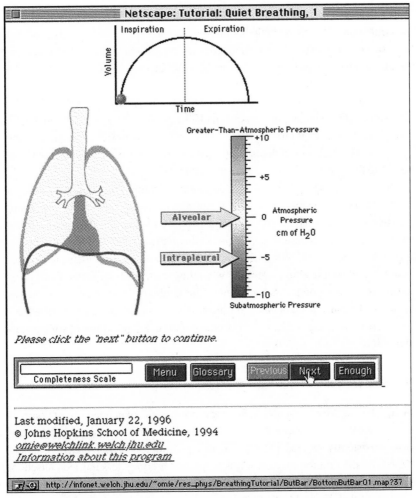

Figure 6.5   A Web page in the Respiratory Physiology tutorial.

In 1995 and 1996, we reimplemented the project for the World Wide Web (http://omie.med.jhmi.edu/res_phys/index.HTML). Figure 6.5 shows a sample page of that site.

A spin-off of this development has been the production of a number of digital videos that are used alone during lectures (e.g., on bronchoscopy [http://omie.med.jhmi.edu/res_phys/Encyclopedia/Airway/Airway.HTML] and the fluoroscopy of normal breathing [http://omie.med.jhmi.edu/res phys/Encyclopedia/Diaphragm/Diaphragm.HTML], both with edited video frames labeled to indicate location and anatomy).

In 1993/94, we attempted to induce students to create a question bank that we could computerize to aid their studying. Despite attractive rewards (students who submitted questions were included in a lottery for three $100 bookstore certificates), we received only two reasonable submissions, and the contest (and the idea) were discontinued.

We used the Internet for several aspects of course administration. In 1993, the course notes that already existed in electronic form were made available on the Welch Medical Library's gopher system. Also in that year, a "question of the week" was E-mailed to students for discussion. The course notes were later transferred to the LectureLinks Web-based system.

In 1995, we used the InfoNet to create an environment for obtaining student feedback for each lecture and lab in Respiratory Physiology. The system maintains strict anonymity by immediately stripping identifying information from evaluations. In a separate file, it registers the names of the students who evaluate each lecture. Thus, course directors can determine which students have evaluated which lectures but cannot see what they said. We have found that giving extra credit to students who complete the evaluations is the most effective method of ensuring feedback. The incentives provided in other courses have been less motivating and have produced precipitously lower rates of student participation.[5]

Support for Other First-Year Courses

While the majority of faculty members supported the expanded use of computers in education, this was not true of all. The Biochemistry senior faculty members consistently showed no interest in using computers in their area and, at first, expressed the opinion that there was no place for computers in medical school teaching. However, the junior faculty showed increasing interest.

The Molecules and Cells faculty have been much more accommodating. In 1995, the course director made a commitment to putting lecture notes on-line (and, in fact, was the first to do so) and to using the Web-based lecture evaluation system. Unfortunately, because the evaluation system was neither mandatory nor exclusive (paper evaluation forms were also used), almost no students used this system. Also in 1995, the Histology image database was expanded for use during the histology portion of Molecules and Cells.

The Anatomy course has used a number of external on-line sources since 1993, primarily the illustrated anatomy atlas A.D.A.M.® In 1995, OMIE developed a digitized, labeled video of the pelvis, using the National Library of Medicine's Visible Human Male data (Spitzer, Ackerman, and Scherzinger 1996).

This video was important not only in teaching the pelvis but also in making students aware of the Visible Human Project, an important national informatics project.

The Developmental Biology faculty have been interested in computer material because of the students' difficulties in grasping embryonic development. In 1993, we helped the National Library of Medicine evaluate its computer program Cardiac Embryology, which was developed at the Audiovisual Program and Development Branch of the Lister Hill National Center for Biomedical Communications. The program, based on the Carnegie Collection of Human Embryos (housed at the Human Development Anatomy Center at the Armed Forces Institute of Pathology), was made available for Johns Hopkins students. The faculty also suggested that students use MacBaby®, a commercially available program. In 1994, we added EmbryoImage®. Finally, as part of our NEMSC collaboration, in 1994 we were able to make the Basic Embryology Review Program (developed by the University of Pennsylvania) available for Johns Hopkins students. Faculty members used some of the digitized videos in their lectures.

In 1995, we expanded the use of the Histology image database to the Immunology course. The Neuroscience faculty have used a number of new programs quite successfully: Stanford University's Brainstorm, New York University's Brain Slices, and the University of Washington's Digital Anatomist are prime tools, as is our local Weigert-stain image project, developed by Dr. Mark Molliver. All of these have been used annually since 1993.

Support for Second-Year Courses

We directed less effort toward second-year courses, primarily because there were not enough computers even if we had been able to motivate the faculty. Our strategy was to lead students to want computer support in the hope that they would demand it from the second-year faculty. This strategy worked to some extent; during the summer of 1995 a first-year student circulated a petition that garnered forty signatures asking for more computers. This request was one factor in the decision to expand the IRC computer lab. In 1996, when the director of the second-year curriculum retired, he was replaced by a faculty member who had a strong interest in using computers in the second-year curriculum.

The Cardiology, Pulmonology, and Pathology faculty have expressed the most interest in computer-aided instruction for the second year. Our support for Cardiology consisted of finding an adequate tutorial on EKGs; we chose ECG-on-Disc®. For Pulmonology we re-presented the Respiratory Physiology tutorial that we had developed for the first year. For Pathology, we provided students with the Virgil image-based teaching program, which was developed at Vanderbilt University.

Support for the Clinical Years

No education-oriented computers are available to students in the clinical years beyond those in the IRC. The Internal Medicine Clerkship used a patient simulation program called CBX (Clauser et al. 1993) for teaching, but that project was stopped for administrative reasons.

Nevertheless, we have pursued a number of projects for the clinical years. Primary among these was developing an on-line case simulation environment for the required Neurology Clerkship (George et al. 1996). The goals of case simulation are to teach history taking and neurological examination, with secondary goals of teaching imaging interpretation and the appreciation of differences among presentations of various types of "opathies." The specification document for the project pointed out that because of the variability of students' exposure to important disorders, the scattering of students to various learning sites, and the deficiencies of current evaluation methods vis a vis clinical disorders, students needed standardized exposure to a common set of patient presentations in a manner that would enable evaluation of students' thinking, not just of their responses to multiple-choice questions. Although clinical simulations with standardized patients would be ideal, computer-based simulations are a close second. We selected a commercially available case-development "shell" called DxR® (Myers and Dorsey 1994) for creating cases. DxR includes a didactic model of what the student should learn and a model to be used by faculty to critique the student's decisions; these are the program's main strengths. Using a shell allowed us to focus on the process of creating cases rather than on programming itself. It took six months to create the specifications for the project and to select the shell, another few months to organize the people in the project, and another six months to develop the first case. The project required a total of twenty hours of faculty time and thirty hours of student time (George et al. 1996). In the spring of 1996, the case we developed and two others that we purchased became a required part of every student's learning and formative evaluation in the Neurology Clerkship. Students found the simulation helpful but insisted that their performance on simulated cases not be used as a formal part of their summative evaluation by the faculty.

Our other efforts for the clinical years have concentrated on the information infrastructure as a whole. For example, to further our goal of ubiquitous and continuous access to educational materials, OMIE worked with the Division of Biomedical Information Sciences and the Johns Hopkins Hospital to develop specifications for the hospital's desktop computers. The specifications anticipated student needs for computer applications that eventually would become available to hospital personnel on the wards, and determined the form in which educational material would be made available to students in the hospital. In collaboration with Dr. Kevin Johnson of the Department of Pediatrics (who represented the Information Services Organization in this project), Dr. Barbara Frink, the director of nursing systems and research at the hospital, and others, we conducted a paper survey of medical students, residents, and nurses. Students and house staff gave almost identical responses. The respondents were asked to rank their levels of interest in eighteen possible uses for computers. They expressed the greatest interest in computer use for direct patient care (discharge summaries, lab test results, and patient scheduling), for viewing radiographs, for literature searching, and for faxing to referring physicians. Radiograph viewing and faxing were not supported at the time of the survey.

The net result of this effort was that the hospital, with some medical school funding, placed two Windows-based machines and a printer in every clinical unit. These machines support the hospital information system, the locally developed Electronic Patient Record, and the World Wide Web browser Netscape Navigator. The hospital's commitment to supporting Internet access was a major step toward the realization of our vision of providing Internet-based, just-in-time learning during the clinical years.

Students' Reactions

While some faculty members have been slow to accept educational technology, the students have been uniformly enthusiastic. In a student-run survey of the first-year classes in 1992 and 1993, computer resources were rated as one of the best parts of the curriculum, including the old curriculum at a time when computer development was limited to the efforts of the Neuroscience faculty.

In response to a 1994 survey, first-year students in the second iteration of the new curriculum reported that, on a scale of 1 to 5, they valued computer-aided instruction (average rating of 3.88) second only to lectures (4.79), and higher than the 1993 students did ($3.58, p < 0.05$), a change that reflected our increased activity. In 1995, 78 percent of the class of 1997 and 79 percent of the class of 1998 signed a statement of goals for the new curriculum, one of which was to "encourage computer-aided instruction as a supplement to other methods of study."

Medical Informatics Results

Our development of a plan for curriculumwide training in medical informatics proceeded in three steps: (1) creating a list of desired learning objectives in medical informatics; (2) determining where in the current curriculum those objectives were already satisfied; and (3) determining how to satisfy the remaining objectives.

Medical Informatics Learning Objectives

For step 1, Karla Hahn (then the Internet librarian) and I worked out the conceptual framework according to which medical informatics needs would be defined. Starting with the classic definition of medical informatics (Shortliffe et al. 1990), we divided informatics into four dimensions: functionality, enabling knowledge, knowledge of methods, and tools. Functionality, in turn, breaks down into high- and low-level functions. High-level functions are the purposes that information management is supposed to serve: patient management, education (teaching and learning), research, and practice management. Low-level functions are those needed to accomplish these purposes: data collection, data organization, data analysis, communication, and security. To be proficient in all of these functions, physicians must have a core understanding of the underlying principles (enabling knowledge), must be aware of the ways in which enabling knowledge can be applied (methods), and must be skilled in using the hardware and software that put the methods into action (tools). Appendix 6.2 outlines these dimensions. Many efforts associated with medical informatics focus on tools rather than function levels, knowledge, or methods.[6]

For step 2, we attempted to perform a paper-based survey of course directors. The questionnaire (app. 6.3) was based on the conceptual framework just described. Unfortunately, the response rate was lower than 30 percent, and we were unable to generalize from the responses we did receive.

The faculty were not ready for an organized distributed curriculum, and we were left to rely on grass-roots efforts. For example, the faculty committee that was designing the Generalist Clerkship, which became the Ambulatory Clerkship in Internal Medicine, was very receptive and included informatics education (Internet access, decision-making systems, and expert systems) in their course design. In addition, our proposed Literature Searching Practicum was instituted, and time was made available in the curriculum to teach students about computer-based patient records before their clinical rotations.

Appendix 6.3 shows how the current four-year curriculum satisfies the informatics learning objectives (see column 4). Note that many of our objectives turn out to be satisfied in the current curriculum.

Literature Searching Practicum

The one major informatics intervention in the curriculum was the Literature Searching Practicum.[7] The ability to search the medical literature on-line is viewed by all medical educators as an essential skill (Shelstad and Clevenger 1994; Blonde, Goldstein, and Guthrie 1991; Guyatt et al. 1992). The Welch Medical Library has taught this skill in many ways for many years, but medical students did not take the classes offered by the library, either because of schedule conflicts or because the classes were not part of the old curriculum. In 1993, the Committee for Computers in the Curriculum successfully introduced a requirement that first-year medical students demonstrate proficiency in literature searching.

Dr. Kerryn Brandt, the library's program director of information management and curriculum support, who was also an assistant professor in the Division of Biomedical Information Sciences, was primarily responsible for the content. We have published an account of our experience with the practicum (Brandt and Lehmann 1995). The current course content is available at http://www.welch.jhu.edu/classes/tut/lit-srch/.

The core elements of the practicum are (1) a didactic component; (2) a research project (students create a bibliography based on a question they formulate); and (3) a quiz on which students must score 40 percent or higher to pass. Students may place out of the didactic component by demonstrating prior knowledge; however, fewer than 10 percent do so.

The didactic component is a two-hour session with a small group of students (ten or fewer) and one faculty member (Dr. Brandt or Dr. Lehmann). In 1993, the first year of the practicum, we linked the practicum to a clinical correlation, expecting that the correlation would stimulate questions. This link was not successful and was dropped. Also in 1993, we had faculty subject-matter experts review the bibliographies for face validity. (Did the students catch the known important articles?) This review delayed feedback to students by many weeks and afforded them little additional learning. It was dropped, in favor of review by the teaching faculty. Initially, we required the practicum students as a group to generate a single bibliography that would be distributed to the rest of the class. We thought that students would be more motivated if they were creating a resource for other students, but this incentive was not motivating, and it, too, was dropped. It took a few years of experimenting with ideas to achieve what we, and the students, believe to be a worthwhile experience.

Electronic Patient Record

As is shown in our framework for informatics functions (app. 6.2), the computer-based patient record is a key tool for implementing various medical informatics concepts. The Johns Hopkins Hospital has instituted an Electronic Patient Record project (known as EPR '95) that is currently implemented in the pediatric and medical outpatient clinics and eventually will be used throughout the hospital. A full description of it is beyond the scope of this chapter.[8]

Conclusions

Our experience in relation to the four operating principles discussed previously can be summarized as follows:

1. *Computer software can help students acquire the knowledge they need for clinical decision making.* A core assumption of medical education is that knowledge of basic science translates into better decision making in the clinical years. We have put that assumption into practice by creating LectureLinks as a reminder and reference system, based on the World Wide Web. The Neurology case simulation and the terminated CBX program were classic efforts in computer-based clinical decision making, and we plan to extend those experiences.[9]

2. *A collaborative, networked computer environment is essential for modeling the multidisciplinary clinical activities in which students will later take part.* This principle is at the heart of the network plan described earlier and in figure 6.2. With a network services group that understands the Internet and with the commitment of the Division of Biomedical Information Sciences to provide educational material on-line, students can look forward to a future of network-based computing.

3. *A medical informatics curriculum can help to prepare students for the clinical world.* The Literature Searching Practicum was the first informatics course ever required of Johns Hopkins students and, in fact, the first requirement that they demonstrate any level of competence in that area. The degree to which we have succeeded in other areas of the informatics curriculum is summarized in column 4 of appendix 6.3.

4. *Researching new informatics methods and investigating the effectiveness of informatics activities in medical education are integral components of success in the use of informatics in the curriculum.* Thus far, our research has focused on the Web-based materials we developed, which we have evaluated primarily by means of surveys of students before, during, and after their use of the software. Further evaluations are planned.[10]

It was suggested earlier that medical informatics would have an impact on six objectives of the education reform project. The extent of that impact is reviewed in the following sections.

Computerizing Learning and Teaching

Gene E. Hall and Shirley M. Hord (1989), in their writings about the process of instituting change in medical schools, note five phases of faculty response: ignorance, fear, interest, use, and advanced use.

We encountered a fair amount of faculty ignorance, apathy, and even fear of computers. The shortage of computers for the students aggravated this problem; limited access to the available computers made it difficult to entice even those faculty members who were interested. As faculty members have become aware of our services, they have approached us, saying, "Why haven't we heard of you before? You shouldn't rely on the course directors to spread the word!" The LectureLinks project is the easiest way of involving and accommodating these faculty members, many of whom are lecturers. We have been fortunate in having a number of champions on the faculty who appreciate and enjoy the use of computers in education. The Physiology and Histology faculties have been particularly enthusiastic supporters. At the same time, some faculty have done well on their computers without any help from us. This pleases us, although some have let their eagerness get in the way of a systematic approach to software development.

Rewarding Faculty for Teaching

Even for faculty who want to produce educational materials for the students, the lack of rewards has proved to be a particularly frustrating barrier. We have tried to carve out faculty time through internal grants. One faculty member's attempt at earning external funding through the NIH for a computer-based education curriculum in a medical subspecialty failed only because, according to the evaluation sheets, the principal investigator (also a faculty member) was judged as being too junior by the NIH study section concerned.[11]

Expanding the Use of Case-Based, Small-Group Learning Sessions

We purchased large-screen computer monitors in part because they would enable students to work together. Our anecdotal observations confirm that students do their computer-based learning in pairs about half the time. We would like to integrate computers into faculty-led small groups, but again, the lack of hardware at this point is a major obstacle.

Integrating the Basic Sciences with Clinical Experience

The need to integrate knowledge of basic science with clinical experience is one of the reasons for the creation of LectureLinks. With a networked computer resource, clinical clerks can consult basic science lecture notes on-line as reminders and can access Web-based material for primary learning.

Expanding Ambulatory Experiences

With the Neurology case simulation project, we hope to provide the first of many "virtual" experiences in ambulatory medicine. We have also worked with the Ambulatory Clerkship in Internal Medicine to bring evidence-based reasoning to bear in clinical decision making.

Incorporating Social Issues into the Study of Medicine

Several informatics topics are under consideration for inclusion in the Physician and Society course.

Summary

Our experience in introducing computers into the curriculum confirms Thomas Edison's observation that invention is 10 percent inspiration and 90 percent perspiration. We are aware that other schools have used similar methods, some with better and some with worse results. If we have achieved success, it is due to three sets of people. First is the high-quality OMIE staff. Second is the Welch Medical Library staff. With their true service orientation, they have taken risks and expended resources that no one else would have. Third are Dr. Kingsbury and his staff. Their effort in centering the Johns Hopkins information services on the network has enabled us to move forward with our vision of network-based learning.

From the outset, there was tension between our goals of delivering educational technology to the students and teaching them medical informatics concepts. There were a number of reasons for this tension. First, because the curriculum was already under stress from the curtailment of hours in well-established courses and the addition of a new four-year course (Physician and Society), we felt that adding an explicit educational objective and new course of our own would be too invasive. Second, there was a history at Johns Hopkins of disappointment with computers because of the perceived failure of a cutting-edge clinical information system in the mid-1980s. Third, to most faculty members, "informatics" meant computers, not the intellectual foundations of computer-based information systems. These issues all posed challenges that we still face.

There is no doubt that informatics in general, and computers in particular, will become more important to the practice of medicine. As managed care organizations limit the number of days physicians can take off for education, as continuing medical education moves to the Internet, as medical records move to computers, students will find that much of medical thought and practice is based on informatics principles and takes place through computers. This electronic revolution has arrived at just the moment when educators are reconfiguring the curricula of medical schools across the United States and elsewhere. We hope that the informatics concepts and the computer-based tools that our students master while at Johns Hopkins will enable them to continue their education in this brave new world.

Appendix 6.1 Educational Technology Framework and Schedule for 1995

COURSE	Faculty development	Acquisition	Development	Integration	Delivery
Year 1					
Molecules and Cells	Supporting faculty as needed	Outlining images Review of Histology electron micrographs Scanning of images	Developing lab image database from individual images Database review	Creating handouts for the database	Making database available Teaching and supporting users
Anatomy	Determining which videos would be most useful		Creating digital videos from Visible Human data: Getting appropriate data Creating video	Integrating digital videos into course/lectures Creating handouts	In-class demo Teaching students and faculty to use the videos Loading videos to server and user units Continuing use of A.D.A.M. and other software Making CD-ROM available
Developmental Biology	Determining which parts of available software are useful			Revising instructional handouts	Teaching faculty to use the videos Loading movies to lecture computer Loading IRC software to work-stations

Immunology	Supporting faculty	Completing the image database	Integrating the database into course/lectures Editing database contents (done during Molecules and Cells)	Loading database to the server and user units
Neuroscience	Verifying that available software is still appropriate		Editing handouts	Loading software to workstations Making CD-ROM available Ensuring that some machines are available during lab time
Physiology		Surfactant tutorial Verifying MacLung (computer-based laboratory) Transferring Interactive Respiratory Physiology to the Web Creating surfactant tutorial Obtaining art from students	Helping users in respiratory simulation lab Revising instructional handouts	Supporting cardiac and respiratory physiology simulation labs Loading software to workstations

(continued)

157

Appendix 6.1 (*continued*)

COURSE	Faculty development	Acquistion	Development	Integration	Delivery
Histology	Supporting faculty as needed	Finding replacement images	Maintaining image database; Working with new image set (electron micrographs)	Ensuring compatibility with lab sections; Auditing content of image database	Loading software to server and to workstations; Ensuring that some machines are available during lab time
Literature-Searching Practicum					
Physician and Society			Modifying course content	Creating schedule from record of student log-ins	Teaching the course; Supporting E-mail-based essays
Clinical Epidemiology	Meeting with faculty, developing specifications	Helping in the selection and purchase of statistical software		Creating handouts; Creating data sets for teaching	In-class demo; Teaching and supporting users; Loading software to workstations
Year 2					
Pathology		Reviewing Vanderbilt images			Loading software to workstations; Teaching users

Pharmacology					
Microbiology	Developing specifications	Finding ancillary software	Customizing software	Creating instructional handout	Loading software to workstations
Physician and Society					
Clinical Years					
Neurology and Psychiatry	Teaching faculty about case-simulation software	Working with DxR staff Simulated-case creation	Making case simulation part of Neurology Clerkship formative evaluation	Scoring user performances Loading software to workstations Ensuring confidentiality of results	
Projects					
Software purchasing	Needs assessment	Choosing possible software candidates from database Acquiring software evaluation copies	Performing evaluations Customizing software	Creating instructional handout	Loading software to workstations
LectureLinks	Getting all course directors (five per quarter) involved in providing lecture notes and publicizing resource availability	Finding remote Web sites and reviewing with faculty Collecting material from course administrators Miscellaneous paper scanning	Regenerating LectureLinks each quarter Creating LectureLinks database on InfoNet Marking up lecture notes Modifying LectureLinks database	Reviewing Web sites with faculty and students for propriety	Maintaining the LectureLinks environment Managing user requests

(continued)

Appendix 6.1 (*continued*)

COURSE	Faculty development	Acquistion	Development	Integration	Delivery
Sofware database Overlayer			Adding entries and culling outdated entries Adding advanced questionnaire functionality		
Access			Creating environment that uses Welchlink accounts as security to workstations		Loading Access software and consistent version of AtEase® on all workstations Standardizing user environments Fixing bugs Supporting users
InfoNet-based lecture/lab evaluations	Obtaining faculty consent to perform evaluations	Obtaining schedules Obtaining modification to questionnaires Modifying questionnaire Distributing questionnaire Data input	Modifying InfoNet	Interacting with course administrators	
Computer survey of incoming students			Analyzing data and writing report		

160

Appendix 6.2   Informatics Fuctions

Information Function	Knowledge and Methods	Tools
Patient Management		
Collect data	Take history and perform physical examination, gather lab and imaging data, create differential diagnosis	CPR,[a] diagnostic expert system, image recognition system
Take action	Select test, choose therapy	Decision support systems, expert systems
Communicate action	Order tests or therapy, record decisions	Physician's worksheet, electronic order-entry system, CPR, spoken and written interaction, health smart card, telemedicine
Education (Teaching and Learning)		
Collect data (learning)	Search research literature, find appropriate course	Electronic library databases and search software, CPR
Collect data (teaching)	Determine the audience knowledge profile	Instant-tally devices and software
Take action (learning)	Read literature, learn material	Full-text bibliographic databases, CAI[b]
Take action (teaching)	Write article, compose presentation, give presentation, create CAI	Productivity tools (office suites), authoring software
Communicate action (learning)	Demonstrate knowledge, demonstrate attendance	Computer-based tests, electronic CME[c] registration
Communicate action (teaching)	Document teaching activities	Electronic CME registration and database
Research		
Collect data	Collect research data	CPR, electronic data forms
Take action	Analyze data, design study	Statistical packages, statistical expert systems

(continued)

Appendix 6.2   *(continued)*

Information Function	Knowledge and Methods	Tools
Communicate action	Report results	Productivity tools, Internet
Practice Management		
Collect data	Determing case-mix, cash flow, and case-based performance	CPR, accounting software, clinical practice guidelines
Take action	Create marketing strategy, choose business practices, implement continuous quality improvement	Forecasting software, management decision-support systems
Communicate action	Perform marketing, collect receivables, interact with regulatory agencies	Business software, Internet

[a]CPR = Computer-based patient record.
[b]CAI = Computer-aided instruction.
[c]CME = Continuing medical education.

Appendix 6.3   Questionnaire for Course Directors.
This questionnaire, based on the framework shown in appendix 6.2, was sent to all course directors. Conclusions are given in the right-hand column.

Medical Informatics Education Objectives across the Curriculum

Name _____ Course _____

Please fill out the following checklist of educational objectives. (1) What priority would you assign the objectives *anywhere* in the curriculum? (Use the following scale: 1 = literature searching [highest], 10 = computer programming [lowest]). (2) Is the objective taught in *your* curriculum? (3) Would you want the objective as a prerequisite to your course? (4) Notes: Please write here if you think the objective should be taught as *part of your course.*

OBJECTIVE	(1) Priority (1 → 10)	(2) Taught	(3) Pre-requi-site	(4) Notes [For puposes of this chapter, this column is used to indicate percentage of students achieving a skill, or the location in the curriculum where the knowledge or skill is taught.]
COMPUTER LITERACY				
Skill in using Graphical User Inerface	❏	○		*At least 80%, by matriculate survey*
Skill in using word processor	❏	○		*100%, by matriculate survey*
Skill in using spread-sheet	❏	○		*17%, by matriculate survey*
Skill in using presenta-tion software	❏	○		
Skill in using a database management system	❏	○		*9%, by matriculate survey*
Skill in using electronic mail	❏	○		*At least 70%, by matriculate survey; probably higher, due to Welchlink*
Knowledge of computer networking	❏	○		

(continued)

Appendix 6.3   *(continued)*

OBJECTIVE	(1) Priority $(1 \rightarrow 10)$	(2) Taught	(3) Prerequisite	(4) Notes [For pupuoses of this chapter, this column is used to indicate percentage of students achieving a skill, or the location in the curriculum where the knowledge or skill is taught.]
Knowledge of basic computer management issues (security, access control, backup)	❑		◯	*Orientation for use of clinical systems at the Johns Hopkins Hospital*
PATIENT MANAGEMENT				
Data Collection				
Knowledge of the structure of medical language	❑		◯	
Knowledge of the structure of medical records	❑		◯	
Knowledge of hospital information systems	❑		◯	*Clinical Skills*
Knowledge of Computer-Based Patient Record	❑		◯	
Skill in using computer-based patient records	❑		◯	*EPR '95[a]*
Skill in using computer-based images	❑		◯	*First-year CAI[b]*
Skill in using image-interpretation software	❑		◯	
Decision Making				
Skill in using diagnostic expert-system software	❑		◯	
Skill in using computer-based clinical practice guidelines	❑		◯	
Skill in using formal decision analysis	❑		◯	
Skill in using a personal database of patient records	❑		◯	*Patient log in Ambulatory Clerkship in Internal Medicine*

(continued)

Appendix 6.3   *(continued)*

OBJECTIVE	(1) Priority $(1 \rightarrow 10)$	(2) Taught	(3) Pre-requi-site	(4) Notes [For puposes of this chapter, this column is used to indicate percentage of students achieving a skill, or the location in the curriculum where the knowledge or skill is taught.]
Skill in using computer-based order entry	❏	○	*SMS Orders system in the Johns Hopkins Hospital*
Knowledge of tele-medicine	❏	○	
LEARNING MANAGEMENT				
Skill in searching reference and full-text databases	❏	○	*Literature Searching Practicum*
Skill in Internet searching	❏	○	*Literature Searching Practicum*
Skill in critical appraisal of the clinical research literature	❏	○	*Clinical Epidemiology, Ambulatory Clerk-ship in Internal Medicine*
Skill in using computer-aided instruction	❏	○	*First-year CAI[b]*
Skill in using computer-network-based material	❏	○	*LectureLinks*
TEACHING MANAGEMENT				
Skill in creating computer-aided instruction software	❏	○	
Skill in creating patient education material	❏	○	
PRACTICE MANAGEMENT				
Knowledge of health microeconomics	❏	○	*Physician and Society*
Knowledge of practice configurations	❏	○	
Knowledge of quality assurance	❏	○	

(continued)

Appendix 6.3 *(continued)*

OBJECTIVE	(1) Priority (1 → 10)	(2) Taught	(3) Pre-requi-site	(4) Notes [For pupuses of this chapter, this column is used to indicate percentage of students achieving a skill, or the location in the curriculum where the knowledge or skill is taught.]
Skill in using appoinment-scheduling software		❏	○	
Knowledge of quality improvement		❏	○	
POLICY MANAGEMENT				
Knowledge of health macroeconomics		❏	○	*Physician and Society*
Skill in critical appraisal of the public health literature		❏	○	*Clinical Epidemiology*
Skill in querying outcomes database		❏	○	
Knowledge of treatment algorithms		❏	○	*Clinical Clerkships*
Knowledge of auditing methods		❏	○	
Skill in managing personnel		❏	○	
Skill in critiquing own or other's guidelines		❏	○	
Knowledge of automated clinical reminders		❏	○	
RESEARCH MANAGEMENT				
Skill in bibliography management		❏	○	
Knowledge of research design		❏	○	*Clinical Epidemiology*
Skill in analyzing data		❏	○	*Clinical Epidemiology*
Skill in using statistical packages		❏	○	*Clinical Epidemiology*

[a]EPR '95 is the name of the computer-based patient record, running on Windows 3.1 client machines.
[b]CAI = computer-aided instruction.

Notes

The author gratefully acknowledges the assistance of Bonnie Cosner, Joan Freedman, Jayne Campbell, Rob Sapp, and David Kingsbury in writing this chapter.

1. Dr. Kingsbury left Johns Hopkins in 1997.

2. The NEMSC was disbanded in 1997; it was made unnecessary by the ease of long-distance collaboration on the Web.

3. In 1997, OMIE developed a standards-based database to support LectureLinks, so that course directors in other divisions and schools could replicate this tool.

4. This program has since been ported to the Web (http://omie.med.jhmi.edu/cvsim4).

5. More recently we performed a randomized crossover trial of paper-based versus Web-based evaluations. Our preliminary analysis indicates that students prefer paper evaluations. Course administrators prefer the Web for logistical reasons.

6. Our framework was adopted by the American Association of Medical Colleges as an important component of the informatics objectives of the association's Medical School Objectives Project.

7. This course is now called the Information Searching Practicum because of its inclusion of the Web and other resources.

8. The project has won the prestigious Computerworld Smithsonian Award for Use of Technology to Benefit Humanity. Further information on the project is available at http://jhmcis.med.jhu.edu/.

9. In 1997, we began developing a Web-based version of a clinical-encounter simulator, based on the Interactive Patient program (http://medicus.marshall.edu/medicus.htm), under the direction of Dr. Christoph Lehmann (no relation to the author).

10. In 1996, we performed a fully factorial crossover evaluation of the impact of making the Histology image database available in the laboratories during lab exercises. The outcome measures were self-report questionnaire responses by students and faculty and observations by an ethnographer. In brief, the results showed that computers were appreciated and filled a useful niche in learning, although the respondents' characterizations of that niche are not easily summarized.

11. The medical school is currently making explicit in its criteria for the promotion of faculty members that development of quality educational materials, including those that are computer-based, will be considered as a positive element of a faculty member's portfolio.

Bibliography

Association of American Medical Colleges. 1992. *ACME-TRI report: Educating medical students.* Washington, D.C.: Association of American Medical Colleges.

Blonde, L., D. Goldstein, and R. D. Guthrie Jr. 1991. "Teaching internal medicine: Using computers in internal medicine education." Ochsner Clinic, Jefferson, La.

Brandt, K. A., and J. M. Campbell. 1995. "Bibliographic instruction plus: A short course in scientific communication for graduate students in the basic sciences." *Medical Reference Services Quarterly* 14:77–85.

Brandt, K. A., and H. P. Lehmann. 1995. "Teaching literature searching in the context of the World Wide Web." *Journal of the American Medical Informatics Association* (Symposium Supplement, Proceedings of the Nineteenth Annual Symposium on Computer Applications in Medical Care) 2:888–92.

Clauser, B. E., et al. 1993. "Factors influencing performance on clinical simulations: Using clinician ratings to model score weights for a computer-based clinical-simulation examination." *Academic Medicine* 68:S64–S66.

De Bliek, R., C. P. Friedman, and E. F. Purcell. 1983. *The new biology and medical education: Merging the biological, information, and cognitive sciences.* New York: Independent Publishers Group.

Dwak, A. R., N. Jurisic, P. Dev, H. M. Hoffman, and A. Irwin. 1994. "CC-IMED: The California Consortium for Informatics in Medical Education and Development." In *Symposium on Computer Applications in Medical Care: Eighteenth annual meeting,* edited by J. G. Ozbolt, 986. Washington, D.C.: Hanley & Belfus.

George, E. B., M. J. L. Eliasson, J. Freedman, and H. P. Lehmann. 1996. "Computerized interactive clinical case presentation: Teaching students to think like neurologists." *Neurology* 46:A117.

Guyatt, G., et al. 1992. "Evidence-based medicine: A new approach to teaching the practice of medicine." *JAMA* 268:2420–25.

Hall, G. E., and S. M. Hord. 1989. *Change in schools: Facilitating the process.* Albany: State University of New York Press.

Learning Resource Center. 1995. *Software for health sciences education: An interactive resource.* 6th ed. Ann Arbor: University of Michigan Medical Center.

Lehmann, H. P. 1995. "The migrations of an image database: Flat file, relational, object." In *Computers in Healthcare Education Symposium: Managing the Information Mosaic,* edited by R. B. Murray, 34. Philadelphia: Thomas Jefferson University.

Lehmann, H. P., and M. R. Wachter. 1995. "Delivering structured educational images over a network." In *Nineteenth Annual Symposium on Computer Applications in Medical Care,* edited by R. M. Gardner, 989. New Orleans: American Medical Informatics Association.

Matheson, N. W., and J. A. Cooper. 1982. "Academic information in the academic health sciences center: Roles for the library in information management." *Journal of Medical Education* 57:1–93.

Mattern, W. D., et al. 1992. "Computer databases of medical school curricula." *Academic Medicine* 67:12–16.

Myers, J. H., and J. K. Dorsey. 1994. "Using diagnostic reasoning (DxR) to teach and evaluate clinical reasoning skills." *Academic Medicine* 69:428–29.

Nowacek, G., G. Miller, and C. Young. 1995. "Curriculum textbase: A faculty resource for instruction." In *Innovations in Medical Education Exhibits: Twentieth annual session,* edited by M. E. Whitcomb, 71. Washington, D.C.: Association of American Medical Colleges.

Shelstad, K. R., and F. W. Clevenger. 1994. "On-line search strategies of third-year medical students: Perception vs. fact." *Journal of Surgical Research* 56:338–44.

Shortliffe, E. H., L. E. Perreault, G. Wiederhold, and L. M. Fagan. 1990. *Medical informatics: Computer applications in health care.* Reading, Mass.: Addison-Wesley.

Spitzer, V., M. J. Ackerman, A. L. Scherzinger, and D. Whitlock. 1996. "The Visible Human Male: A technical report." *Journal of the American Medical Informatics Association* 3:118–30.

Stephens, P. A., and J. M. Campbell. 1995. "Scientific writing and editing: A new role for the library." *Bulletin of the Medical Library Association* 83:478–82.

Stoner, J., and M. Heider. 1995. "A curriculum database at the University of Cincinnati." In Whitcomb, *Innovations in Medical Education Exhibits,* 74.

7

Introduction to Clinical Medicine

Nancy Ryan Lowitt, M.D., Ed.M.,
and Diane M. Becker, Sc.D.

The Concept

With the introduction of the revised four-year curriculum in 1992, the Johns Hopkins University School of Medicine began an ambitious and innovative journey that has substantially altered both the content and the teaching methods of a professional education in medicine. Based on principles of adult learning and designed to promote independent, creative, and integrative thinking and a lifelong interest in learning, the new curriculum challenges students and faculty to define and master a foundation of scientific knowledge within a context or framework that will facilitate an individual learner's acquisition of new information in the months and years of professional life ahead.

This innovative approach is well suited to meeting the challenges of teaching in the clinical medical setting. As the volume of medical information soars and as our ability to capture and access information electronically increases our scientific databases daily, medical practitioners are in need of a firm foundation in clinical sciences, a framework for managing new data, and the skills of personal reflection and interpersonal communication that can bring medical science to the examination room as resource for human beings in a healing partnership. Early experience with community-based practicing physicians was designed to be one of the foundations of the new first-year curriculum. This experience was designed to help students acquire firsthand knowledge of the way a good physician relates to patients by observing their preceptors and by observing themselves and attending to their own feelings in their conversations with patients.

When the Association of American Medical Colleges (AAMC) surveyed the class of 1950 ten years after graduation to determine in which of four general areas of instruction their medical school experience had been most deficient, 42 percent chose "practical instruction in the doctor-patient relationship."[1] There is considerable current interest in studying the nature of this relationship, in identifying the skills that may facilitate successful doctor-patient interactions, and in designing curricula to improve these skills at all levels of training.

Within the structure of our new curriculum are courses in biomedical and behavioral sciences, the four-year Physician and Society course, and a second-year course, Clinical Skills, which includes formal instruction in conducting the medical interview. The first-year Introduction to Clinical Medicine was introduced to round out the doctor-patient-interaction component of the new curriculum. In this course, students are paired with community-based faculty mentors and spend an afternoon every two weeks with them in their practices. At midyear, students change sites so that they can have two different experiences. A portion of the class spends half of the year in a community-based health program (described later in this chapter) rather than with a second physician preceptor. Providers are asked not to expect the students to learn clinical medicine or comprehensive interviewing techniques because these subject areas are addressed in the second-year Clinical Skills course and in the later Ambulatory Clerkship in Internal Medicine. The main aim of Introduction to Clinical Medicine is that the time spent with community-based physicians and their patients should constitute attention to the artful part of medicine, which is, after all, an "artful science" best learned from role models.

Mentoring is a time-honored and traditional method for training in interpersonal skills. Indeed, most respondents in the AAMC survey of the class of 1950 reported learning most about the doctor-patient relationship from observing their instructors.[2] The advantages of mentoring include the strength of the interpersonal relationship that may develop between student and teacher and the opportunity to experience the daily life of a practicing physician through observation.

Introduction to Clinical Medicine was begun in an effort to bring students and practicing physicians together for a mentored clinical experience in settings removed from classrooms and laboratories. In the early years of the new curriculum the course goals, learning objectives, and teaching methods were identified and refined. The new four-year curriculum of the medical school facilitates an expansion of the role of learner to include not only observation (passive and active), but active participation and critical reflection. In Introduction to Clinical Medicine the student, as adult learner, uses all of these approaches to develop a foundation of knowledge for use in the clinical setting and a framework for continuing personal and professional growth as a scientist and healer.

Course Director and Preceptors

Finding a course director and a sufficient number of qualified, willing community-based physicians was not easy. Because none of our community-based, part-time faculty had been involved in directing anything like the proposed program, Dr. Catherine De Angelis, vice dean for academic affairs, decided to coordinate it herself for the first year. This would allow time for a leader to emerge from among the physicians who precepted students in their offices. After several months, it became obvious that Dr. Richard Freeman was the front leader, and he became the course director. Dr. Freeman left the program after three years to assume another position, and at that point, Dr. Nancy Lowitt became the director.

The sixty-three physicians who precepted the students in the first year were chosen and personally contracted by Dr. De Angelis. (Chapter 2 gives a fuller explanation of this process.) Because of the natural turnover, each year a number of new preceptors must be found. This ongoing search is one of the responsibilities of the course director, who now personally chooses and contacts potential new preceptors.

Needs Assessment

The needs assessment for this course included focus group discussions with physicians in practice, several members of the Educational Policy Committee, and first-year students. On the basis of priorities identified by the focus groups, the course is designed to enable students to (1) have fun, (2) not be overloaded with paperwork, (3) begin the process of professional socialization through immersion in practice and role-modeling, and (4) possibly develop long-term friendships with their preceptors.

The physicians in practice urged that we emphasize the study of the helping relationship, the development of interviewing skills for eliciting the "patient's side of the story" and conveying empathy, personal and intellectual growth of the future physician, and specific content areas important to primary care, such as ethics and economics. Students, initially unsure of what they should learn in a course like this, were nonetheless eager to begin working with patients and with their clinical mentors early in the first year. Students' concerns initially centered on time constraints and potential competing demands from other courses in the first year. This essentially proved not to be a problem.

Goals and Objectives

Three fundamental goals for Introduction to Clinical Medicine were developed from discussions and literature reviews, using a perspective that placed the course in the context of a broad four-year curriculum. The goals, and the educational objectives that define them, are included in the course syllabus for students to review with their preceptors.

To define the goals and help students and preceptors attain them, specific educational objectives have been defined for each. To help students develop an understanding of what it means to be a practicing physician, they are asked to focus on the *goals* and *objectives* of the program. These are as follows:

Goal 1:   To develop an understanding of what it means to be a practicing physician.

Objectives: 1:1 To learn how physicians meld several skills—developing a relationship with the patient, gathering clinical data, and applying clinical reasoning and medical knowledge—in the medical encounter.

1:2 To learn how physicians manage time, their office staff, and themselves in order to care for their patients and to provide time for themselves, including time for maintenance of professional competency.

1:3 To establish personal learning goals in consultation with the preceptor.

This goal and these objectives help students develop a clearer view of the practicing physician by identifying the skills they may need to nurture and balance the many components of their personal and professional lives.

Goal 2:   To develop a basic understanding of the patient-physician relationship.

Objectives: 2:1 To develop the sensitivity and skills needed to elicit from patients their experience of illness.

2:2 To begin to learn to respond to particular concerns of a particular patient at a particular time.

This goal and these objectives help students develop an understanding of the special responsibilities and relationships of the practicing physician.

Goal 3:   To develop an early awareness of professional identity.

Objectives: 3:1 To understand what it means to be a doctor in a helping relationship.

3:2 To describe to fellow students and preceptors one's emotional responses to encounters with patients.

All of the above-cited goals and objectives broadly highlight skills that are
later taught explicitly in the medical interviewing component of the second-year
Clinical Skills course and other courses such as Physician and Society. Students
in Introduction to Clinical Medicine are not taught how to conduct a comprehensive interview, but rather are asked to observe, practice, and reflect on communication skills they use daily to build rapport, trust, and understanding. These
skills can be viewed as tools necessary to fostering successful physician-patient
relationships.

Teaching Methods

The prescribed teaching methods for Introduction to Clinical Medicine are intended to promote active, self-directed learning skills consistent with the principles of adult professional learning. The conceptual methods are experiential
learning, promotion and acceptance of the student as a novice professional, emphasis on comprehension rather than rote learning, and a close working relationship with a mentor who can help students plan and carry out individualized
learning plans.

Concretely, preceptors and students are advised to review a menu of educational activities that address course objectives and to consider choosing activities from it. They are also asked initially to review, together, a list of guidelines
for student participation in the clinical encounter so that the students will feel
free to participate actively as is appropriate. The course guide suggests planning
activities in a chronological order that is coordinated with the content of the larger concurrent first-year curriculum, so that the various components may be experienced as part of a coherent whole.

Early in the year, from September through November, students are advised
to focus on development of the sensitivity and skills needed to elicit a patient's
experience of illness, awareness of their emotional responses to patients, and the
establishment of personal learning goals in consultation with the preceptor.
These objectives build on students' natural curiosity and personal responses to
the intimate nature of patients' stories. Students may participate in clinical encounters as they work on these objectives. During this time students are also taking the Molecules and Cells course (which includes biochemistry, cell biology,

molecular biology, genetics, and immunology). Concurrently, the Physician and Society course introduces the history of medicine, including topics such as the craft, profession, and science of medicine, and the decline of the country doctor.

Activities introduced at this time of the year include those that serve the above-mentioned objective of developing the sensitivity and skills needed to elicit patients' experience of illness. The student observes patient interviews and examinations conducted by the preceptor; maintains a log that lists, for each patient observed, the issues, problems, and concerns elicited during the interview; discusses with his or her preceptor (at the end of each session) some of the issues noted in the log and reflects on why these are important to the patient at this point in his or her life; and reads appropriate components of the course guide as well as a suggested text.

Later in the semester, students may wish to speak with patients about their experience of illness, present their findings to the preceptor, and obtain feedback from the patients and/or the preceptor on the skills used during the interview. To develop awareness of their emotional responses to patients and colleagues, at the end of each day the students discuss with the preceptor both their own and the preceptor's responses to certain patients or colleagues.

After the third or fourth session, the student meets with the preceptor for the purpose of developing personal learning goals. The student then reflects on what has been most meaningful so far and what would be the most fun to pursue, given the real limitations of competing demands on both the preceptor's and the student's time and the nature of the practice. For example, preventive care might be of special interest to the student. The preceptor can offer a practical overview, provide appropriate literature to the student, and involve the student in discussing clinical guidelines for preventive care for each patient.

During the middle third of the year, approximately from December through February, students are engrossed in Anatomy, Developmental Biology, and some of the following topics in Physician and Society: medical ethics, truth telling, confidentiality, and cross-cultural issues in medicine. In Introduction to Clinical Medicine during this period, the focus is on the course objectives of understanding what it means to be a doctor in a helping relationship and learning how physicians manage time and balance personal and professional demands. Also, during this time period, students change office sites for the second half of the precepting program and have an opportunity to reflect on differences between the two experiences.

To enable students to understand more fully what it means to be a doctor in a helping relationship, we suggest that the preceptors take an active role in making explicit the skills they use to forge compassionate, ethical relationships with their patients. For example, during the clinic session they may discuss with students what current biomedical technology can offer a particular patient and how they use available evidence to rank options for care, which they then discuss with patients. Or discussion at the end of the day may focus on how the helping relationship and care of the patient continue even when "there's nothing more to do" for the patient with a terminal illness.

To learn how physicians manage time, their office staffs, and themselves, students are urged to spend time with the preceptor's staff to learn how they have been organized as an efficient team of providers. Students and preceptors are encouraged to discuss the balance of professional life with other personal priorities, the process of identifying those priorities, and the process of negotiating balance.

In the last part of the year, students are encouraged to focus on the two remaining objectives: learning to respond to the concerns of a particular patient at a particular time, and learning how skilled clinicians meld development of doctor-patient relationships, clinical reasoning, and medical knowledge in the medical encounter. These high-order, integrative objectives are most readily attained on the basis of the preceding objectives and, like them, are supported by the content of concurrent courses, including organ physiology and histology, neuroscience, and behavioral science. Topics covered in Physician and Society during this time include health economics, communication in medicine, and other management issues in medicine.

To further the objective of learning to respond to the particular concerns of a particular patient, preceptors can choose either to observe a student's discussion with a patient and offer feedback, or to review the student's log entries on a particular patient. Preceptors and students are urged to consider alternative responses to challenging moments in interviews, and to reflect on how the interviews might have gone differently as a result.

To make explicit the reasoning processes and skills physicians use—in particular, those involved in melding development of doctor-patient relationships, clinical reasoning, and medical knowledge in the medical encounter—preceptors are asked to discuss the process through which they have arrived at a diagnosis for a particular patient. What questions were raised by the patient's chief complaint? How did the preceptor know what to ask next? A discussion of relevant syllabus articles might enhance this discussion.

In summary, preceptors and students are offered opportunities for action and reflection in exploring the nature and depth of the doctor-patient relationship. Specific skills can enhance the attainment of the educational objectives of the course, and the faculty and students are offered suggestions for developing these skills through defined activities, although it is recognized that much learning will occur in the unique and unpredictable moments of a clinical practice day.

Community-Based Health: Introduction to Cultural Issues in the Practice of Medicine

With the initiation of the new curriculum, it was recognized that exposure solely to traditional office-based practices in medicine may omit learning experiences in high-risk communities with highly specific cultural needs.[3] Dr. Diane M. Becker, the founder of a community health care partnership between the Johns Hopkins medical school and the East Baltimore community, designed and piloted an innovative program for first-year medical students using experiential empowerment (i.e., "working together to make a difference"). Health care delivery systems are making a shift toward community care, which will have a major impact on the way that physicians are trained to practice medicine.[4] Currently, groups at the greatest risk for serious chronic and infectious diseases and populations with needs for improved preventive health services are often seen only at the time of an acute illness or at a later stage of diagnosis. In the future, physicians' training will better prepare them to deal effectively with such situations and to provide preventive services.

The basic elements of a good doctor-patient relationship—communication and trust—are more difficult to achieve when there is discordance between the cultures of the physician and the patient.

Yet unique cultural needs that interact with the practice of medicine in the community often are not addressed in medical school. Not surprisingly, therefore, few young physicians choose to practice medicine with poor and low-income populations.[5] This occurs despite the fact that many underserved populations are located in urban areas literally in the shadows of large academic medical centers like Johns Hopkins.[6] In these centers, local urban communities tend to be highly represented among the patients seen by medical students and residents.

The Johns Hopkins University School of Medicine is located in an inner city community that is primarily African American. Many African Americans in the community work at the hospital and use it as their main source of care. Still, relationships with the medical care system are variable. Misuse of emergency facilities for chronic or acute minor illnesses is common. To help medical students learn how to address some of the unique aspects of working with this community, a twelve-week component in community medicine (extending over one-half year) was added to Introduction to Clinical Medicine and piloted for three years. The overall goal was to provide students with a context for understanding the diversity of patient needs in an environment of competing social, economic, and cultural pressures. Piloting and evaluation began in the 1993/94 academic year. Selected students spent one of the two semesters of Introduction to Clinical Medicine in the community health program. At the end of 1996 we temporarily suspended the program in order to reassess our resources and goals; we then made a plan to reinstate the program, and a second pilot was begun in January 1998. This chapter describes the first phase, from 1993 to 1996.

Objectives of the Community Health Program

After the first year, on the basis of feedback from students and community preceptors, the objectives of the community health program became more explicitly focused on communication between care providers and patients. The revised objectives, implemented in the second and third years, were to

1. provide a repertoire for adapting communication and implementation of medical practice to different populations;
2. provide a context for understanding social and cultural factors in health and illness from a community perspective; and
3. expose students to real-world community experiences.

The course offered an opportunity for first-year students to be introduced to the care of whole communities and to work as part of multicultural and multidisciplinary teams.

Community Health Field Placements

For the twelve weeks of the community medicine component of Introduction to Clinical Medicine, students attended four-hour field placements weekly in the local community. Their preceptors included physicians and nurses in community health centers, neighborhood health workers, teachers and social workers in school-based programs, social service professionals, and outreach personnel in settings such as Health Care for the Homeless. A course coordinator monitored all field placements through regular contact with the field preceptors and through on-site visits with the students.

Students often chose to spend more than four hours per week in field placements. Many organized independent projects. For example, two students working in a school-based asthma clinic designed an afternoon jump-rope club for asthmatic children to improve exercise capacity and the ability to manage symptoms during exercise and play. The program is now operated by parents and teachers in one of the largest elementary schools in the United States. Another student designed a nutrition and fitness program for patients in an AIDS care facility to improve their quality of life. One student assisted a local community organizer, who was a preceptor for the course, in initiating a HUD program that integrated health education with job training for adolescents. Together they sought and were awarded a $1 million, five-year grant to provide job training and health care for high-risk urban youth. The emphasis in all of these extracurricular projects and in the basic field experience was empowerment rather than "doing for."

The extracurricular projects were self-initiated. Most students enjoyed the field placement, although not all of them put in extra time. A few were disappointed; these individuals generally wished for a more traditional clinical placement.

Student Selection for the Community Health Program

Although the Introduction to Clinical Medicine course was mandatory, only half of the class participated in the community health pilot program, which was optional. Forty-two percent of the class indicated that they had engaged in community service in the past, but only 15 percent had any sustained or intensive experience.

For the first year of the pilot, only students with records indicating a strong background in community health were assigned to the program. This group was almost uniformly committed to community health work. For the second year, students were chosen purely at random. For the third year, students were sent a questionnaire during the preceding summer assessing their interest, and only students who rated the community medicine experience highly were selected.

Students were offered an annotated list of potential field placements and then were interviewed by the course coordinator to select an appropriate host site. One field placement was with the forensic pediatricians in the Child Advocacy Network, who dealt with children who were being treated for abuse and neglect. Students at this site were required to integrate the physician-patient interaction with family counseling and exposure to the law enforcement and justice systems. Other field placements, such as the East Baltimore Medical Clinic, part of a local HMO, provided students with an experience of more traditional outpatient care, supplemented by home visits in the company of physician preceptors. In general, the more interactive a student was with the site preceptor, the more successful the field experience. Field preceptors were selected from among individuals known to the course director. Most had a history of mentoring medical and nursing students in outpatient community sites.

Seminars on Culture and Health

The community health program included ninety-minute, semimonthly seminars on culture and health. These were facilitated by a medical school faculty member engaged in community-based medicine and a local community leader (often a pastor) with training in multicultural community care.

Discussions in the seminars were student-directed. Half of the time was reserved for discussion of students' experiences in the field placements, half for discussion of videos and readings. Usually one component or the other dominated. Group sizes ranged from eight to fifteen students. The smaller groups interacted more comfortably. Students often helped one another with problems at their field sites. Occasionally, a whole group would come together for an extra, student-organized seminar, at which the "organizing" students would present a "case" from their own site for discussion. Each semester, John Singleton's *Boyz N the Hood* and videos of the speeches of the Reverend Dr. Martin Luther King Jr. were popular discussion topics. Students expressed a desire for more multimedia experiences like these.

Because each seminar was offered twice, students who missed a session were asked to make it up. Missed field experiences were also made up, at the negotiated convenience of the preceptor and student.

Readings and Supplementary Resources

A combination of health care literature and popular literature was selected for the community health program by a team of medical school faculty, students, and instructors from the community. James Baldwin's *Fire Next Time* was required reading.[7] It was used to stimulate discussion of the difficulties encountered by medical staff in melding the perspectives of two very different cultures. Reference texts and selected articles addressing multicultural health issues were also required reading. We created a manual of contemporary readings, to be updated each semester. Three texts on African American health were used as references.[8]

"Insider" tours of the Johns Hopkins Hospital, conducted by hospital employees in nutrition, housekeeping, security, and support services, were offered as elective experiences to give students a local community perspective on the hospital. Relevant theater and multicultural opportunities were offered free of charge.

Evaluation of the Community Health Program

The evaluation of the Community Health Program was based on questionnaires administered to students before and after the course. The responses were grouped by numbers that represented the individual test takers, who were not identified by name in the output. After data entry, the master list of names and numbers was destroyed. Students knew that this part of the evaluation was anonymous. The range of sociodemographic and community experience that students brought to the program were the same in the second and third years of the pilot, independent of the ways the students were selected. Therefore, the evaluation was administered to all 107 students.

To assess students' knowledge and attitudes about culture and health, we performed a literature review and developed a questionnaire. The questionnaire was piloted, then was administered before and after the course only in the second and third years of the program.[9] Included were questions on the social demographics of students, prior community experience, experience with other cultures, beliefs and attitudes about other cultures, and knowledge about general health problems in underserved urban populations. There was little variance in responses. The majority of students had little or no knowledge of African American culture and openly indicated the fact. On average, in response to each of six questions about social customs in the African American community, 71 percent of the students answered "don't know."

The proportion of students who expressed concern about their ability to relate to people of different cultures in the doctor-patient relationship and who expressed social or physical fear of working in community settings was noted at baseline to be 60 percent. This is not surprising given the homogeneity of the students' lifestyles before entering medical school. Most came from suburban or rural backgrounds (81%) and predominantly white secondary schools (52%), and had attended undergraduate programs in Ivy League colleges (48%) or small white liberal arts colleges (14%). Demographically, 43 percent of the participants were European American, 33.3 percent Asian American, and 19 percent African American; 85.8 percent were science majors and 48 percent were female.

The majority of students were unable to estimate correctly the relative importance of chronic diseases, substance abuse, teen pregnancy, and violence in the urban environment. Most indicated that the major causes of morbidity and mortality, independent of age, were homicide, substance abuse, alcohol abuse, and poor health practices. The responses represented traditional myths about the nature and distribution of health issues in the urban community. Although the African American students, for the most part, had backgrounds similar to those of the rest of the class, they found the culture and belief questions to be offensive because of their stereotypical nature. At posttest, 85 percent of the students indicated a marked change in their opinions about inner city culture and a greater willingness to explore options to improve the doctor-patient relationship and communication. Most of the remaining 15 percent indicated that they had been comfortable at the outset and hadn't needed to adjust their opinions.

Most of the students indicated that the combination of field placements and seminars was influential. Some even indicated that this had been a life-changing experience. Lectures and readings were rated much lower. Films, theater trips, hospital tours, and elective adjuncts were rated highly, although only 50 percent of students participated.

When asked if they would take this course again, nearly 95 percent of the 107 students who participated indicated that they would do so, with few or no changes. The remaining students felt that the time commitment was too great or that the course material was biased. A group of six students in the final pilot year lobbied for a more aggressive approach to race and racism as a major issue in health care.

A definite shift occurred in questionnaire responses, which indicated that students experienced a greater degree of comfort with the local community and with unfamiliar cultures after the course. Just before the course, 63 percent of the students had indicated that poor community residents placed a very low value on personal or family health; after the course, only 30 percent expressed this opinion. (Before and after the course, 24 and 15 percent, respectively, answered "don't know" on this item.) Before the course, 71 percent saw cultural differences as a barrier to health care in underserved urban communities; only 43 percent held this opinion after the course. It is possible that social desirability bias was responsible for this shift; however, students had been informed that the questionnaires would not be viewed by instructors and that the data would be examined in the aggregate only.

Written Requirements

All students in the community health program completed a five-page synthesis paper at the end of the twelve weeks. They were free to choose any style and content for the assignment. Some papers were deeply personal and indicated a major change of perspective on the concept of "helping." Some were traditionally scholarly and referenced, with discussions of the required academic readings. Others were simple descriptions of what students had done during the course, with no interpretation. Students also kept a weekly subjective journal of their field experiences, to be shared with the instructors. Finally, each student was required to write a discussion of his or her "case" or special project from any perspective. The papers were not graded but were used simply to enhance student self-awareness and to cue faculty in helping students in their personal and professional development. All materials were returned and were viewed as the personal property of the student.

Future Plans

Today, as the new community health pilot program evolves, faculty, students, and community members continue to evaluate the program and to consider various possible configurations. The question of how to fully integrate the program into Introduction to Clinical Medicine is particularly challenging, given the sociopolitical nature of the experience.

The community health program requires a major faculty time commitment. Directing and participating in the program requires at least a 25 percent effort by a senior faculty member. Additional faculty participate at about 10 percent effort in a faculty-student ratio of 1 to 32 over the course of the academic year. Community leaders (1 to every 32 students) also devote four to six hours per week to teaching and planning. A course coordinator is necessary to assign students to the field, monitor students and field preceptors, organize seminars and electives, and assist in data collection for ongoing evaluation of the course. Field preceptors participate without pay or other incentives. The majority commit their time voluntarily and are welcoming to students. This is a labor-intensive course for both the teaching team and the students.

The ramifications of field work and seminars located in the community and partially mentored by community workers are noteworthy, for individual students and for the field of medicine as a whole. It is important to involve community perspectives in designing an appropriate curriculum that has physician education as its primary goal. The community medicine program has served as the springboard for many students to explore nontraditional career options that address the needs of high-risk populations. In an era of change in the medical care structure, the emergence of leaders in community-based medical care is crucial to the development of a sensitive and responsive health care system.[10]

Evaluation of Introduction to Clinical Medicine

Evaluation of the Introduction to Clinical Medicine course, including field placements through the community health program and in private physician offices, occurs continuously and involves formative and summative evaluation methods.

The course in its entirety is examined by the school of medicine and the AAMC as part of the comprehensive evaluation plan for the first-year curriculum. The focus of this evaluation is the expectation that the course meet the stated goals for the new curriculum of promoting approximate attitudes, values, knowledge, and skills that will form the foundation for lifelong learning. Within the structure of the first year and throughout the four-year curriculum, early and increased exposure to clinical medicine in mentored ambulatory settings has been identified as a means of promoting the development of skills in humanistic clinical medicine. The goal of the first-year experience is for the student to gain firsthand knowledge of the way a good physician relates to patients. (Specific, standardized training in the conduct of patient interviews and physical examinations occurs later in the curriculum, as does specific teaching of evidence-based medical practice and decision making.) This summative evaluation process in the context of the general curriculum is described elsewhere.

Student satisfaction with this course is assessed in formative and summative ways. Formative evaluation—that which is collected during the course and can influence midcourse changes where needed—occurs both informally and formally. Students are quite comfortable about communicating with the course director by electronic mail and are encouraged to use this venue for any feedback they wish to offer. Structured focus groups with students and faculty have been used throughout the four years to identify specific concerns and to develop approaches to address them. Certain current course activities, such as discussion of curricular goals that the course is meant to fulfill, maintenance of patient logs by the students, and the midyear switch of preceptor sites, originated from suggestions by students and faculty. Information from focus groups, from the first-year curriculum committee, and from individuals involved with the community health seminars has also resulted in midcourse changes. Students were an integral part of the process of reassessing the community health program during its temporary period of suspension.

It remains to be seen whether the Introduction to Clinical Medicine course can be isolated as a contributing factor in any of the four general evaluation criteria identified in the initial proposal for the new curriculum: student general satisfaction, student satisfaction with specific courses and programs, performance on course and national exams, and choice of speciality for postgraduate training. Tentative future plans for summative program evaluation include assessing the degree to which this early mentored exploration of the clinical doctor-patient relationship influences student attitudes toward the practice of clinical medicine in the community.

Notes

1. H. H. Gee, "Learning the physician-patient relationship," *JAMA* 173 (1960):1301–4.

2. Ibid.

3. R. Tuckson, "Community-based training: Getting the details right," in *Academic health centers in the managed care environment,* ed. D. Korn, C. J. McLaughlin, and M. Osterweis (Washington, D.C.: Association of Academic Health Centers, 1995).

4. Council on Graduate Medical Education, *Managed health care: Implications for the physician workforce and medical education, sixth report* (Washington, D.C.: USDHHS, HRSA, 1996); and Bureau of Health Professions, *The education of generalist physicians: State of the art conference compendium* (Washington, D.C.: USDHHS, HRSA, 1993).

5. M. E. Whitcomb et al., *Impact of federal funding for primary care medical edu-*

cation on medical student choices and practice locations, (Washington, D.C.: HRSA, Office of Rural Health Policy, 1991).

6. D. M. Levine et al., "Community–academic health center partnerships for underserved minority populations," *JAMA* 272 (1994):309–11.

7. J. Baldwin, *The fire next time,* 4th ed. (New York: Random House, 1991).

8. W. L. Reed, W. Darity, and N. L. Roberson, *Health and medical care of African Americans* (Westport, Conn.: Auburn House, 1993); E. J. Bailey, *Urban African American health care* (Lanham, Md.: University Press of America, 1991); and M. G. Secundy, ed., *Trials, tribulations, and celebrations: African American perspectives on health, illness, aging, and loss* (Yarmouth, Maine: Intercultural Press, 1992).

9. N. Warfield-Coppock, "Toward a theory of Afrocentric organizations," *Journal of Black Psychology* 21 (1995):30–48; and H. Landrine, "The African American acculturation scale: Development, reliability, and validity," *Journal of Black Psychology* 20 (1994):104–27.

10. J. R. Hogness, C. J. McLaughlin, and M. Osterweis, eds., *The university in the urban community,* Sun Valley Forum on National Health (Washington, D.C.: Association of Academic Health Centers, 1995).

Bibliography

Barker, L. R. "Curriculum for ambulatory care training in medical residency." *Journal of General Internal Medicine* 5 (1990; suppl.):S3–14.

Barker, L. R. "Developing a program to teach humanistic medicine: Where in the curriculum?—house staff" Paper presented at Teaching Humanistic Medicine Conference, New York University, November 1989.

Barker, L. R., E. Bartlett, and A. Golden. "The doctor-patient relationship: Communication and patient education." In *Principles of ambulatory medicine,* edited by L. R. Barker, J. Burton, and P. Zieve, 30–41. Baltimore: Williams & Wilkins, 1995.

Barrows, H. S. "Problem-based, self-directed learning." *JAMA* 250 (1983):3077–80.

Barsky, A. "Hidden reasons some patients visit doctors." *Annals of Internal Medicine* 94 (1981):492–98.

Beckman, H., and R. Frankel. "The effect of physician behavior on the collection of data." *Annals of Internal Medicine* 101 (1984):692–96.

Branch, W. T. "Doctors as 'healers': Striving to reach our potential." *Journal of General Internal Medicine* 2 (1987):356–59.

Branch, W. T., et al. "Teaching medicine as a human experience: A patient-doctor relationship course for faculty and first-year students." *Annals of Internal Medicine* 114 (1991):482–89.

Cassel, E. "The nature of suffering and the goals of medicine." *New England Journal of Medicine* 306 (1982):639–45.

Emanuel, E. J., and L. L. Emanuel. "Four models of the physician-patient relationship." *JAMA* 267 (1992):2221–26.

Enelow, A., and S. Swisher. *Interviewing and patient care.* New York: Oxford University Press, 1986.

Kahn, G. S., B. Cohen, and H. Jason. "The teaching of interpersonal skills in U.S. medical schools." *Journal of Medical Education* 54 (1979):29–35.

Kassirer, J., and G. Gory. "Clinical problem solving: A behavioral analysis." *Annals of Internal Medicine* 89 (1978):245–55.

Kay, J. "Terminating the doctor-patient relationship." *Journal of Medical Education* 53 (1978):186–90.

Kern, D. E., et al. "Residency training in interviewing skills and the psychosocial domain of medical practice." *Journal of General Internal Medicine* 4 (1989):421–31.

LaCombe, M. "Point of view: The doctor." *Americal Journal of Medicine* 85 (1988):404.

Lazare, A. "Shame and humiliation in the medical encounter." *Archives of Internal Medicine* 147 (1987):1653–58.

McCue, J. "The effects of stress on physicians and their medical practice." *New England Journal of Medicine* 306 (1982):458–63.

Monahan, D. J., et al. "Evaluation of a communication skills course for second-year medical students." *Journal of Medical Education* (1983):372–78.

Neufield, V. R., and H. S. Barrows. "The 'McMaster philosophy': An approach to medical education." *Journal of Medical Education* 49 (1974):1040–50.

Novack, D. H., C. Dube, and M. G. Goldstein. "Teaching medical interviewing: A basic course on interviewing and the physician-patient relationship." *Archives of Internal Medicine* 152 (1992):1814–20.

Olmsted, A. G., and M. A. Paget. "Some theoretical issues in professional socialization." *Journal of Medical Education* 44 (1969):663–69.

Quill, T., and P. Townsend. "Bad news: Delivery, dialogue, and dilemmas." *Archives of Internal Medicine* 151 (1991):463–68.

Rabin, D. "Compounding the ordeal of ALS: Isolation from my fellow physicians." *New England Journal of Medicine* 307 (1982):506–9.

Sheehan, T. J., et al. "Teaching humanistic behavior." *Teaching and Learning in Medicine* 1 (1989):82–84.

Smith, R., and R. Hoppe, "The patient's story: Integrating the patient- and physician-centered approaches to interviewing." *Annals of Internal Medicine* 115 (1991):470–77.

Taylor, W. C., R. J. Pels, and R. S. Lawrence. "A first-year problem-based curriculum in health promotion and disease prevention." *Academic Medicine* 64 (1989):673–77.

Yonke, A., and R. P. Foley. "Overview of recent literature on undergraduate ambulatory care education and a framework for future planning." *Academic Medicine* 66 (1991):750–55.

8

Curriculum Reform
in the Clinical Years

H. Franklin Herlong, M.D.,
Patricia A. Thomas, M.D., F.A.C.P.,
and John H. Shatzer, Ph.D.

Changing the Clinical Curriculum

The Johns Hopkins clinical curriculum builds on the strong background of basic medical sciences that students acquire in their first two years. In the final quarter of the second year and the eight quarters of the third and fourth years, each
student follows a clinical educational program adapted to his or her individual
interests and needs. The program includes the required clinical clerkships and
the electives. Students may choose, within certain limits, the order in which they
pursue this instruction. All required clerkships must be taken at the Johns Hopkins Hospital or an affiliated hospital. One quarter of the required elective time
may be taken at another approved institution.

Reevaluating the Required Clinical Clerkships

During the 1994 academic year, the Educational Policy Committee (EPC)
reevaluated each of the required clinical clerkships. The committee's goals were
to (1) collect basic data about the content and scope of all the basic clinical clerkships and formulate goals and objectives for each clerkship; (2) identify objectives and goals common to all the basic clerkships; (3) coordinate the content of
the various required clinical clerkships in such a manner as to meet the future
challenges of medical student education; and (4) address specific topics related
to all clerkships, such as evaluations of the clerkships, disciplinary and peda-
gogic problems with students, and the acquisition of teaching skills by the fac-

Table 8.1 Duration of Clerkships

	Before 1994	After 1994
Emergency Medicine		4 weeks
General Surgery	9 weeks	9 weeks
Pediatrics	9 weeks	9 weeks
Psychiatry/Neurology/Ophthalmology	9 weeks	9 weeks
Obstetrics and Gynecology	6 weeks	6 weeks
Internal Medicine	9 weeks	9 weeks
Ambulatory Internal Medicine		3 weeks
Elective clerkships	39 weeks	32 weeks

ulty. The following summarizes the outcomes of the discussions involving the required clinical clerkships (table 8.1).

Basic Clerkship in Emergency Medicine

The Department of Emergency Medicine requested the creation of a required basic clerkship in emergency medicine. The director of this new clerkship proposed a four-week required rotation based in the emergency department of the Johns Hopkins Hospital. The proposal was approved by the EPC and, subsequently, by the Advisory Board of the Medical Faculty.

During the clerkship, students are assigned four-hour shifts with direct patient encounters in the emergency department. Each day, one hour is devoted to a lecture series. Students are required to keep a log for every patient seen, in which they record presenting signs and symptoms, discharge diagnoses, disposition, and comments concerning follow-up. This clerkship can be taken throughout the academic year and has no prerequisites. Before 1994, the emergency medicine experience was incorporated into the basic clerkship in general surgery. Each student spent two weeks in the emergency department. With adoption of the required Emergency Medicine Clerkship, the two-week emergency department experience in the General Surgery Clerkship was discontinued.

Basic Clerkship in General Surgery

The General Surgery Clerkship is conducted at the Johns Hopkins Hospital, the Johns Hopkins Bayview Medical Center, and Sinai Hospital of Baltimore. During this nine-week experience, students spend four weeks on a general surgery service. With the re-allocation of the emergency department experience to the Emergency Medicine Clerkship, time became available in the General Surgery Clerkship for an additional surgery subspecialty elective. Students select two subspecialty rotations from the following: thoracic surgery, neuro-surgery, plastic surgery, orthopedic surgery, urology, otolaryngology, cardiac surgery, pediatric surgery, and transplant surgery. They also spend one session each week with a faculty member in a general surgery clinic. A daily lecture series provides instruction on various topics in general surgery; a two-hour subspecialty lecture is given three times a week. Small groups, consisting of five students each, meet with surgical preceptors once a week. The course director of the General Surgery Clerkship requested no additional changes.

Basic Clerkship in Pediatrics

The required Pediatrics Clerkship is a nine-week rotation based in the Children's Medical and Surgical Center of the Johns Hopkins Hospital, the Kennedy Krieger Institute for Handicapped Children, the Johns Hopkins Bayview Medical Center, and Sinai Hospital of Baltimore. In some quarters, students rotate through the Union Memorial Hospital, another hospital affiliated with the Johns Hopkins Medical Institutions. The Pediatrics Clerkship includes four weeks of inpatient pediatrics and four weeks of ambulatory pediatric instruction. The ambulatory rotations use the pediatric emergency room, the Harriet Lane Outpatient Clinic, the Kennedy Krieger Institute for Children with Developmental Disabilities, and outpatient clinics at affiliated hospitals. The course director of the pediatric rotation requested no changes in the traditional clerkship.

Basic Clerkships in Psychiatry, Neurology, and Ophthalmology

The clinical clerkships in psychiatry and neurology build on the second-year introductory courses in behavioral science and neurology. In an effort to establish an integrated teaching experience in the clinical specialties related to the nervous system, a quarter-long clerkship program combining psychiatry and neurology is offered. This program consists of four and a half days of ophthalmology, a four-week experience on the psychiatry service, and a four-week experience in neurology. A weekly lecture series and a weekly clinical conference series, each extending over the full eight weeks of the clerkships in psychiatry and neurology, are provided by the psychiatry and neurology departments.

Student assignments in psychiatry at the Johns Hopkins Hospital include the psychiatry units of the Phipps In-Patient Service, Adolescent Psychiatry, General Hospital Psychiatry, the General Psychiatry Consult Service, and the Day Hospital. Students may also rotate through the Johns Hopkins Bayview Medical Center. During the four weeks on psychiatry, students attend weekly grand rounds and three emergency room assignments. Students also rotate through a Sexual Behavior Consultation Unit that is part of the Johns Hopkins Hospital system. The inpatient experience includes daily rounds, patient evaluations, treatment conferences, and teaching rounds.

The four-week neurology rotation also includes an integrated lecture series, along with a comprehensive approach to the diagnosis and management of neurologic disorders. The clerkship stresses skills such as history taking for neurologic symptoms, performance of detailed neurologic examinations, and recognition of normal and abnormal physical findings. Students are expected to learn about the natural history of major neurologic diseases and to develop an understanding of neurologic diagnostic tests, which includes knowledge of neuroradiologic procedures and neurophysiologic tests and the ability to interpret lumbar puncture results.

During the clerkship, students rotate through the inpatient general neurology service and daily outpatient clinics. During the four-week rotation, they participate in a series of case discussions focused on major groups of neurologic diseases, including movement disorders, headache, infectious diseases, dementia, neuromuscular disorders, and epilepsy.

Basic Clerkship in Obstetrics and Gynecology

The Obstetrics and Gynecology Clerkship is a six-week rotation at one of four hospitals: the Johns Hopkins Hospital, the Johns Hopkins Bayview Medical Center, Franklin Square Hospital, or Sinai Hospital of Baltimore. Until 1991, the rotation was a four-week clerkship emphasizing obstetrics, with a two-week course in gynecology and neonatology integrated with the Pediatrics Clerkship. In 1991, obstetrics and gynecology were combined into a six-week clinical rotation.

Each week, three days are devoted to didactic sessions covering basic areas in obstetrics and gynecology. One afternoon each week, a group of students from each site prepares and presents an obstetrics and gynecologic case to a faculty member; this is followed by a clinically oriented discussion of differential diagnosis, evaluation, and management. Among the required conferences are grand rounds and an ethics conference.

Each student receives a syllabus of readings. The syllabus covers important concepts in the field of obstetrics and gynecology, divided into basic areas with subtopics, and presented in the form of case studies. It is meant to serve as a guide for independent study. These clinical case studies are not used in the evaluation of the student. Students use them as a study aid by answering questions provided on the syllabus, after reading the required texts and other references available in the departmental library.

Each student is assigned a faculty preceptor, who should be available to assist the student throughout the clerkship. Students are required to meet with the preceptor at least twice during the six-week program. In this clerkship, the student is considered an integral part of the clinical team and is responsible for directed clinical management. The general goals of the clerkship are to (1) provide an understanding and appreciation of the role of the obstetrician-gynecologist as a primary care provider for women; (2) impress upon students the importance of the gynecologic history and physical examination; and (3) teach basic skills in the overall assessment of the health of women.

Basic Clerkship in Internal Medicine

The Internal Medicine Clerkship is a nine-week rotation conducted in the inpatient units of the Johns Hopkins Hospital, the Johns Hopkins Bayview Medical Center, and Sinai Hospital of Baltimore. Each student spends four and a half weeks in one of the four medical firms at the Johns Hopkins Hospital and four weeks at either the Bayview campus or Sinai Hospital. Four to five students are assigned to a general medical unit staffed by two residents and four interns. The physician of record for patients at the Johns Hopkins Hospital is the assistant chief of service responsible for all patients in the firm.

Department of Medicine faculty serve as physicians of record at both Sinai Hospital and the Bayview campus. Lecture series and small-group discussions complement the inpatient-based clinical instruction. Attending rounds are held three times a week by visiting faculty (these faculty do not have physician-of-record responsibilities).

The course director of the Internal Medicine Clerkship requested an additional four weeks for an ambulatory experience integrated into the clerkship. Fulfillment of this request was postponed until a separate ambulatory experience could be developed.

Initial Proposal for a Generalist Clerkship

In the 1994 academic year, the EPC considered the issue of generalist training and appointed a subcommittee to develop a proposal for a generalist clerkship for medical students. This concept had previously been endorsed by the department directors at a dean's retreat on the curriculum in 1993. The subcommittee included representatives from the departments of Obstetrics and Gynecology, Medicine, and Pediatrics at Johns Hopkins; and the Department of Family Medicine at the affiliated Franklin Square Hospital.

The subcommittee sought to define the ideal generalist clerkship experience, fully recognizing that many potential barriers existed. It was important to the subcommittee that in final form this clerkship attain the same level of excellence as all other required clerkships at the school of medicine. The subcommittee submitted the following proposal (adapted for purposes of this chapter):

GOALS OF THE CLERKSHIP

The clerkship should provide an experience that

1. enables students to participate in the provision of comprehensive, continuing, and coordinated care of patients;
2. develops students' knowledge base about commonly encountered problems in the general care of patients;
3. enables students to incorporate preventive health care into the general care of patients;
4. allows students to serve as the first health care providers to see patients seeking comprehensive and continuing care; and
5. informs the career choices of students.

CLERKSHIP ACTIVITIES

Students would do the initial assessments of new and return ambulatory patients in exam rooms dedicated to student use. Supervision of students would be provided by fellows and faculty in medicine, pediatrics, and gynecology. Family medicine could be recruited from other institutions as well.

Students would act as the patient's primary physician, as if the student were a subintern. Students would be expected to formulate diagnostic and therapeutic plans, provide preventive health care services, coordinate consultative care, provide patient education, and provide or participate in follow-up care. Students would be responsible for all record-keeping.

Organized learning sessions would emphasize self-directed learning through case conferences, morning reports, journal clubs, formal talks, and "case of the week" tutorials. Self-instruction via information systems would be emphasized. Gaps in patient care experiences would be addressed by computer simulation or other simulation exercises. Students would enhance their skills pertinent to general patient care (e.g., skills in the areas of otolaryngology, orthopedics, ophthalmology, dermatology, and psychiatry) through specialty-sponsored activities and through tutorials in effective communication and advanced physical diagnosis.

INSTRUCTORS

Patient care supervision would be provided by faculty and fellows in general internal medicine, general pediatrics, and general gynecology. It also could be provided, under appropriate agreements, by family practitioners from local institutions. The supervisor-to-student ratio would range from 1:2 to 1:3.

The structured learning experiences would rely on faculty from many departments and units. For example, additional instructors could be recruited from otolaryngology, orthopedics, dermatology, and ophthalmology, and from the sexually transmitted disease unit and the AIDS unit. Nursing, nutrition, and social services staff could also be used where appropriate.

PATIENTS

The patients seen on the clerkship could be people of any age, socioeconomic group, or referral source who seek continuing general medical care. These patients would have a variety of reasons for seeking health care, such as assessment of acute, chronic, or multiple illnesses; assessment of general health status; and preventive health screening. Patients would be recruited from a variety of sources, including the emergency room, the Johns Hopkins Referral Service, and links with community health programs.

CONTENT

Each of the goals enumerated earlier determines the content areas appropriate for this clerkship. Obviously, the patient care experiences would provide the most powerful content base. To achieve the goals of the clerkship, however, additional content areas would need to be addressed.

Content areas pertinent to the first goal (providing comprehensive, continuing, and coordinated care of patients) include communication skills; decision making that incorporates clinical epidemiology, clinical practice guidelines, and decision models; record-keeping skills; use of health forms; and appropriate use of experts and expert systems.

Content areas related to the second goal (developing students' knowledge base about common problems) include office gynecology, ambulatory medicine, ambulatory pediatrics, family planning, and recognition of psychiatric illnesses by nonpsychiatrists. More important, self-directed learning would be emphasized, and opportunities for students to share their endeavors in self-directed learning would be provided.

Content areas related to the third goal (preventive health care) include nutrition, occupational health, screening, counseling, assessment and intervention for high-risk behaviors, patient education, and the use of alert systems.

Content areas related to the fourth goal (students' having the first contact with patients) include negotiating skills, prioritizing skills, recognition of physician biases, and appropriate use of follow-up care.

The fifth goal (influence on career choices) could generate specific content areas as well. However, the subcommittee recognizes that the most important factor contributing to this goal would be a robust and realistic clinical experience.

PROPOSED FORMAT FOR THE CLERKSHIP

The clerkship would be a required basic clerkship. Its only prerequisite would be completion of the preclinical curriculum. An effort would be made to link some of the clerkship activities to the Physician and Society course, beginning with the first offering of the clerkship. The clerkship would be a nondepartmental, dean's office course.

The clerkship would combine the final three weeks of the quarter occupied by the Gynecology and Obstetrics Clerkship (a six-week program) with the subsequent half quarter to provide a continuous seven-and-a-half-week experience. Students would not be required to take Gyn/Ob and the new clerkship sequentially, although this would be the most efficient use of their clinical curriculum time. As many as twenty-five students would be accommodated five times yearly.

The clerkship would occupy a dedicated single site, or several contiguous sites at the same location, within the Johns Hopkins Medical Institutions. The subcommittee strongly endorses the creation of a practice site specifically designed to accommodate this clerkship. Maintaining stability of patient care providers would require a dedicated supervisory corps of faculty and fellows, supported by physician assistants and appropriate clinical support services such as a student-patient coordinator, a nursing coordinator, and appropriate clinical and medical records coordinators.

An important aim would be to develop patient loyalty to the clinical operation in spite of the fact that the students would be replaced five times yearly. A strong effort would be made to accommodate family units in the clinical operation and to accommodate walkins and urgent visits. Another aim would be to provide consultation services at the site so that students could participate in consultation visits as well.

EVALUATION

Strategies for student evaluation and program evaluation would be developed. As required by the policies of the school of medicine, students would take a final examination and would receive a final grade using the A-to-F grading system. The final examination is not envisioned as being limited to a written, knowledge-based format.

Program evaluation would ensure that the quality of the clerkship is maintained and that the clerkship achieves its intended goals. Faculty development could be included among the evaluation criteria.

CLERKSHIP ADMINISTRATION

A single course director would be named. Because of the interdisciplinary nature of the clerkship, a group of advisors to the course director would be desirable. Both an administrative assistant and a student-patient coordinator are essential for the success of the clerkship. The student-patient coordinator would schedule appointments to ensure that students are assigned consistently to the same patients. The coordinator would also ensure that each patient is seen by the same faculty group on every visit.

The overhead costs (for space and personnel) would be borne jointly by the school of medicine and the hospital.

BARRIERS

This proposal calls for the development of two new major enterprises: a clinical operation and a required clerkship. These would demand a tremendous initial effort on the part of faculty; however, once established, the faculty effort should be comparable to other activities that combine patient care with teaching.

Two major challenges are recruiting patients and maintaining continuity of care. For continuity of care it is critical to maintain stability of health care providers. This can best be accomplished by a committed faculty with assistance from midlevel practitioners.

FACULTY ISSUES

Sufficient numbers of faculty are needed in order to prevent faculty burnout. Sufficient numbers of faculty also are required to allow patients to feel that they have a small group of personal physicians.

The student clinical practice would not necessarily generate sufficient patient care revenues to support the expense of the practice. The costs of the clinical space, clinical personnel, and clerkship administration must be borne by the school of medicine and the hospital.

Two alternatives exist. One is to place students in a variety of off-campus sites in established practices. This would duplicate experiences provided for students in the first year of the curriculum and would not readily allow achievement of the goals previously stated. The other alternative is to use existing hospital clinics at the Johns Hopkins Hospital and affiliated institutions. This alternative, too, would not readily allow achievement of the clerkship goals; moreover, the number of available sites is currently insufficient. The decentralization involved with either of these alternatives would create organizational difficulties, inconsistent student experiences, and major barriers to the structured learning process envisioned by the subcommittee.

This proposal was approved by the EPC but was not adopted, primarily because of the constraints of cost and space. Instead, a three-week clerkship in ambulatory general internal medicine within the Department of Medicine was adopted as an interim step.

Ambulatory Clerkship in Internal Medicine

With the rejection of the proposal for the generalist clerkship, a subcommittee within the Department of Medicine was charged with developing a basic clerkship in ambulatory medicine. The following is a summary of the current clerkship, as it was implemented in the first year with an enrollment of seventy students.

Goals and Objectives

The subcommittee, chaired by Dr. Patricia Thomas of the Department of Internal Medicine, began its deliberations by generating a list of learning goals and objectives for the clerkship, summarized below. (These were similar to the goals and objectives outlined in the *Core Medicine Clerkship Curriculum Guide*, created as a resource package by the Society of General Internal Medicine and the Clerkship Directors in Internal Medicine.[1] This document also served as a guideline for the clerkship's curriculum development.)

1. Develop core generalist competencies:
   a. care of the healthy patient and preventive medicine;
   b. care of the patient with acute illnesses;
   c. longitudinal care of the patient with chronic illnesses; and
   d. care through a complete illness (especially if chronologically linked to the basic clerkship in medicine).
2. Learn to think like an internist, with emphasis on
   a. diagnostic decision making;
   b. evidence-based, cost-effective medicine; and
   c. self-directed learning.
3. Develop the skills of an internist:
   a. effective communication with patients (developing psychosocial skills, involving patients in decision making, working with cultural diversity);
   b. effective communication with colleagues and ability to work in teams;
   c. comprehensive approach to patient care; and
   d. skills useful in office practice, including urinalysis, minor surgical procedures, pelvic exam, arthrocentesis, and joint and bursae injection.
4. Work with mentors to cultivate
   a. ethical care of patients;
   b. lifelong learning skills; and
   c. balance of professional responsibilities.

Curriculum and Methods

The Ambulatory Clerkship in Internal medicine is a three-week longitudinal block offered in each quarter, accommodating thirty students per quarter. There are no prerequisites for this clerkship. When possible, students can dovetail it with the six-week Obstetrics and Gynecology Clerkship, thereby completing an entire nine-week quarter.

The goals of the clerkship are accomplished through the educational strategies of patient-based learning, small-group learning, and self-directed learning. The patient-based learning experience occurs in five half-day sessions with community-based preceptors in internal medicine practices. At the start of the clerkship, each student completes a personal learning plan with three goals for the rotation, which is shared with the community preceptor. Patients are assigned to students at the discretion of the preceptor, who is oriented to the goals of the curriculum and aware of the student's particular interests. Students are encouraged to see a minimum of two patients per session independently and then to discuss these encounters in depth with the preceptor; the students may see the remainder of their patients by shadowing the preceptor. Each student keeps a log of all patient encounters; to date, these logs have recorded an average of forty-seven encounters per student for the three-week clerkship. The office-based outpatient experience has generated exposure to a spectrum of problems, including the examination of healthy patients and the care of patients with acute illnesses and chronic conditions.

Small-group learning occurs in six two-hour seminars. Groups of five to seven students meet with faculty facilitators for in-depth discussions of disease-based problems such as hypertension and diabetes. The groups also discuss skills pertinent to ambulatory medicine, such as counseling patients to alter health behaviors, conducting a focused medical interview, and using an evidence-based approach in diagnostic evaluations. These sessions are designed to be highly interactive and often include role-playing scenarios. Faculty facilitators encourage students to bring examples of their current clinical experiences to the sessions.

Self-directed learning is woven throughout the curriculum. First, students draw up the personal learning plan mentioned earlier. Second, for each patient write-up, students are asked to state what they learned from that patient, what they feel they need to learn more about, and how they will accomplish that. Third, students receive a booklet for the clerkship written by faculty, entitled *Workbook of Ambulatory Training Problems*. The workbook includes twelve common outpatient training problems, presented in brief outline form, with management strategies, clinical practice guidelines when available, and suggested further reading. Each section ends with a set of self-assessment questions. Students are told that the workbook should be completed in its entirety by the end of the clerkship. Finally, each student submits an evidence-based report, an exercise in which the student chooses a clinical question generated by the patient experience and researches evidence for the use of a particular diagnostic or therapeutic intervention (table 8.2). Students are directed not only to traditional textbook references but also to databases and Web sites so that they can develop proficiency in the use of medical informatics to answer clinical questions.

Evaluation

Throughout the clerkship its goals and objectives are monitored frequently. Student evaluations consist of the following components:

Table 8.2 Summary of Evidence-Based Reports Submitted by Students ($N = 66$)

Item of Analysis	Percentage
Topics chosen for report, by frequency	
Treatment of hypercholesteremia	14
Colon cancer screening	11
Hypertension	9
Prostate cancer screening	6
Treatment of diabetes	6
Treatment of osteoporosis	6
Clinical questions generated by students	
Diagnostic intervention	21
Therapeutic intervention	79
Preventive intervention	45
Grade of research design chosen as evidence	
Randomized clinical trials	71
Outcomes chosen to study	
Mortality	19
Morbidity	77
Cost	0
Students effectively applying the study	
to the original question	97
Mean score of checklist items[a]	87

[a]Each student report was evaluated with a checklist of fourteen items representing application of critical analysis of the literature as outlined in the syllabus.

1. review of the student's learning portfolio, which includes
   a. student-developed learning plan,
   b. patient log (the student's record of patient's problems, age, and sex, and the chosen intervention),
   c. three case write-ups and an evidence-based report,
   d. *Workbook of Ambulatory Training Problems* with answers to questions, and
   e. self-assessment of generalist competencies and clinical skills (table 8.3);
2. Faculty Preceptor Evaluation Form; and
3. standardized-patient clinical examination at the end of the clerkship (the examination incorporates four to six training problems that test basic clin-

Table 8.3 Student Self-Assessment on Completion
of the Ambulatory Clerkship in Internal Medicine, 1997

Core Generalist Competency	Mean Rating
Preventive medicine	3.9
Approach to symptoms	4.0
Chronic illnesses	3.8
Hypertension	4.2
Diabetes mellitus	3.8
Thinking like an internist	
Diagnostic decision making	3.8
Evidence-based medicine	3.8
Self-directed learning	4.1
Skill building	
Communication with patients	4.7
Comprehension approach to care	3.9
Office-based skills	3.8
Balance of professional responsibilities	3.3
Ethical care of patients	3.6

Note: Students were asked to rate personal growth and understanding that they gained from the clerkship in the areas listed, by using the following scale: 1 = None, clerkship didn't address; 2 = Somewhat, just touched on; 3 = Fair; 4 = Moderate, reviewed in depth; 5 = Excellent, feel competent.

ical knowledge; the evaluation includes attention to outpatient issues of communication, counseling, compliance).

Students are asked to evaluate the clerkship on the basis of its various elements, such as hospital-based conferences, faculty, preceptors, utility of the *Workbook of Ambulatory Training Problems,* and utility of the learning portfolio. Student evaluations have been incorporated into formative evaluations of the program, and several changes have been made in the content and objectives of individual sessions on the basis of student feedback as well as student performance. To date, students are enthusiastic about the clerkship; 87 percent report that they "would highly recommend the clerkship to a colleague."

Table 8.4 provides examples of the learning objectives, multiple educational methods, and evaluations used in this clerkship.

Community Preceptors

The success of the clerkship resides in the talent and energy of the community-based preceptors who have opened their office practices to the training of

Table 8.4 Ambulatory Clerkship in Medicine: Sample Learning Objectives, Educational Methods, and Evaluations

Learning Objective	Educational Methods	Student Self-Assessment	Objective Assessment
Ambulatory Training Problems			
Preventive medicine	• Office experience • Workbook chapter • Seminar: "Counseling Patients to Alter Health Behaviors"	Mean self-assessment score: 3.9	Standardized patient examination case: Smoking cessation counseling Mean score: 78%
Hypertension	• Office experience • Workbook chapter • Seminar: "Approach to Hypertension"	Mean self-assessment score: 4.2	Standardized patient examination case: Hypertension Mean score: 71%
Core Competencies			
Evidence-based medicine	• Seminar: "Approach to Chest Pain"	Mean self-assessment score: 3.8	Evidence-based report Mean score: 87%
Communication with patients	• Seminar with role-playing: "Three Functions of the Medical Interview" • Readings	Mean self-assessment score: 4.7	Case reports for data-gathering skills Standardized patient examinations: ratings by standardized patients of students' interpersonal skills during the encounter

Note: Self-assessment scores were collated from end-of-rotation surveys. Students were asked to rate personal growth and understanding that they gained from the clerkship in the areas listed, by using the following scale: 1 = None, clerkship didn't address; 2 = Somewhat, just touched on; 3 = Fair; 4 = Moderate, reviewed in depth; 5 = Excellent, feel competent.

medical students. Community preceptors were recruited from the three affiliated hospital sites, Johns Hopkins Hospital, Johns Hopkins Bayview Medical Center, and Sinai Hospital of Baltimore, through the chief of medicine at each hospital. The number of preceptors consistently available averages twenty-four. Preceptors are eligible to apply for a part-time faculty appointment, but no monetary compensation is offered for such appointments. The preceptors are guests at an annual dinner held in their honor, at which the goals and achievements of the clerkship are reviewed, and they receive vouchers for departmental continuing medical education courses.

What has been the preceptor experience with this clerkship? Twenty-three preceptors returned a feedback survey after the first year of the clerkship. Sixty-one percent of these had precepted a student for one session, 30 percent for two sessions. All of the preceptors reported that the experience had been personally rewarding, citing valued aspects such as interpersonal interactions with students (74%), the opportunity to relearn subject matter ("to teach is to learn anew") (74%), assistance with their workload (22%), and faculty status (13%). The preceptors encountered few negative patient reactions to the presence of students; 43 percent said they had rarely encountered negative reactions, and 57 percent had encountered none at all. The preceptors work in a variety of practice settings; 74 percent reported that their practice administration was very supportive of this effort, 22 percent that it was somewhat supportive, 4 percent that it was not at all supportive. The recruitment and retention of community preceptors will continue to be a challenge for the clerkship.

Summary of Clinical Curriculum Reform

The curriculum reform included a reevaluation of the existing required clinical clerkships, which was accomplished through presentations to the Educational Policy Committee by the course directors in each required rotation. A new required Emergency Medicine Clerkship was established, replacing the two-week emergency medicine experience previously located in the required clerkship in general surgery. An additional two-week elective experience in subspecialties of surgery was added to the General Surgery Clerkship. The required clerkships in internal medicine, pediatrics, obstetrics and gynecology, psychiatry, neurology, and ophthalmology remained unchanged.

The concept of generalist training was addressed by a subcommittee of the Educational Policy Committee. Initially, a seven-and-a-half-week intradepartmental clerkship was proposed. Faculty would be from the departments of Pediatrics, Medicine, and Obstetrics and Gynecology at the Johns Hopkins University School of Medicine and from the Department of Family Medicine at the

Franklin Square Hospital. The proposal requested designated clinic space and a faculty-student ratio of 1:3. This proposal was approved but not adopted because of the constraints of cost and space. Instead, the Ambulatory Clerkship in Internal Medicine was adopted. This three-week required rotation is conducted predominantly in the outpatient facilities of the Johns Hopkins Hospital and its affiliates, and in the offices of general internists throughout the city.

The Office of Medical Education Services

Curricular revisions require new teaching strategies to challenge students, student assessment procedures that match the new challenges, and innovative ways of evaluating the impact of the revisions. While creative teaching faculty are abundant in all medical schools, they often lack the required knowledge of educational theory and design, and of the evaluation methods or educational research tools that are used to test new educational practices. In the current health care delivery environment, academic centers may not afford many faculty the opportunity to develop this necessary expertise. Many schools, instead, turn to individuals trained in education, who can offer the teaching faculty a resource for solving educational problems, implementing new teaching programs, and applying appropriate evaluation methods. Typically, a schoolwide office is established that reports to the dean or an associate dean for academic or curricular affairs. This centralized approach helps to ensure fair access to educational resources while distributing the costs of those resources on a schoolwide basis and at the same time addressing quality assurance issues for new educational programs and research initiatives.

At Johns Hopkins, the Office of Medical Education Services (OMES) was created for this purpose. The mission of OMES is to provide educational support and expertise for faculty in the development of instructional tools, assessment methods, and educational research projects. In October 1991, Dr. John Shatzer was hired as the first director of OMES to assist in the design and implementation of an overall evaluation plan for the anticipated new curriculum. His role as director is to share expertise in educational methods and act as a resource for faculty in educational matters. In the latter capacity, OMES serves as a clearinghouse, providing access to other resources and expertise within the Johns Hopkins community and on a regional and national scale, as well. Within the Johns Hopkins Medical Institutions, a number of faculty possess expertise in certain areas of education. However, a central organization was needed to coordinate educational endeavors. It is difficult for faculty seeking assistance to know of all individuals, projects, and other resources that might be helpful to them.

Another role of OMES is to identify new support services and technologies. Until recently, for example, medical faculty who developed multiple-choice examinations were not supported by machine scoring and analysis systems. Often this meant that individual faculty would hand-score tests, subjecting the process to error and prohibiting any practical application of item analysis for purposes of test improvement. Other faculty would seek outside assistance for machine scoring, creating unnecessary costs of course operation. To fulfill a need that had been identified in several courses, OMES created a scoring and analysis service to assist faculty who use multiple-choice tests.

A third function of OMES is to disseminate Johns Hopkins educational innovations to other institutions and to the medical educational community at large. This has been accomplished in several ways. First, as research and development are implemented, findings are presented in medical education forums. Traditionally, these forums include regional and national meetings and medical education journals; medical school consortia now play a major role as well. As OMES director, Dr. Shatzer has been instrumental in the organization and development of the Baltimore/Washington Consortium of Medical Schools. This consortium consists of the six medical schools in the Baltimore and Washington, D.C., areas, including Johns Hopkins, the University of Maryland, Georgetown University, George Washington University, Howard University, and the Uniformed Services University of Health Sciences. While this consortium has been focused primarily on the dissemination of standardized patient technology, the meetings afford members the opportunity to share other ideas and concerns about medical education issues. Another valuable forum is a national consortium of thirteen private medical schools that meets twice a year. In addition to Johns Hopkins, the Thirteen School Consortium represents Yale University, Harvard University, the University of Rochester, Columbia University, Cornell University, the University of Pittsburgh, the University of Pennsylvania, Duke University, Case Western Reserve University, the University of Chicago, Washington University, and Stanford University. Originally, the consortium was conceived as a platform for discussions among various offices within these schools, including admissions, financial aid, and student affairs; however, as more offices of medical education took part, the need to meet formally as a separate group within the consortium became apparent. Since 1994, each medical school has sent a representative to the meetings. National and local concerns are discussed, new ideas shared, and research agendas developed for joint implementation. Recently, for example, members have implemented a consortiumwide pilot study to examine the clerkship experiences of their medical students in primary care and specialty outpatient care settings. The dissemination of ideas is further enhanced by on-line communications: electronic mail and listservers established to promote dialogue between interested medical education faculty and other health education professionals (e.g., dental education faculty).

These forums help sustain a vibrant and dynamic curriculum, and keep faculty well informed and interested in medical education innovations, principles, and practices.

Another important role of OMES is to provide faculty development opportunities that introduce new methods of teaching and evaluation consistent with intended curricular revisions. This is accomplished in two ways. OMES staff offer internal faculty development sessions in the course of implementing new technologies (e.g., they have taught faculty to use the standardized patient technology for instruction and assessment) and when departments request training for their faculties. Alternatively, OMES brings in experts from other institutions to conduct workshops. This introduces our faculty to new perspectives from other leaders in medical education. The workshops often catalyze new ideas and discussions regarding critical educational issues, ultimately leading to sound educational decisions.

The Clinical Education Center

The Clinical Education Center was created in 1992 to fill the need for a central facility to support clinical teaching, learning, and evaluation for students, faculty, and researchers. When the new buildings for basic science and preclinical teaching were constructed, they included wet and dry laboratories, small-group rooms, state-of-the-art lecture halls, and an Instructional Resource Center, all integral to the design of the buildings. These have been well supported and upgraded as part of the overall educational mission of the school. By contrast, the clinical education sites were scattered throughout the medical institutions. This was due, in part, to the nature of clinical teaching, which is departmentally based and occurs where the patient is treated in the hospital or clinic. Clinical faculty, however, identified a need for an additional hospital space dedicated to the teaching of basic clinical skills and to the support of other coordinated clinical education programs. The faculty's recommendations were ambitious—the center they envisioned would include a large lecture hall, small-group rooms, and an equipped teaching clinic—but hospital space and financial resources precluded such major renovations and purchases. It was decided that an existing area within the Johns Hopkins Hospital could be used, a solution that would minimize the need for renovations.

In 1992, space was secured for the Clinical Education Center within an area that had served previously as the outpatient clinic for digestive diseases (fig. 8.1).

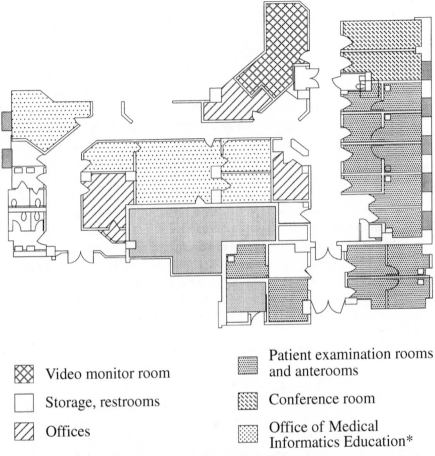

⊠ Video monitor room

▢ Storage, restrooms

▨ Offices

▦ Patient examination rooms and anterooms

▩ Conference room

▥ Office of Medical Informatics Education*

Figure 8.1   The Clinical Education Center is designed for student, resident, and faculty learning, assessment, and educational research. It occupies about 3,000 square feet in the Johns Hopkins Hospital and can accommodate as many as twelve clinical stations, depending on project requirements. There are nine fully dedicated patient examination rooms; six of these have anterooms where students may do additional work, such as post-encounter assessments. All exam rooms are equipped with television cameras and microphones. The video monitoring room is equipped with television monitors and video recorders for observation and recording of the learner's or examinee's performance.

*For information about the Office of Medical Informatics Education, see chapter 6.

A gift from the Johns Hopkins Women's Board provided a portion of the funding that was necessary for minor renovation and the purchase of teaching equipment.

Concurrent with the creation of this facility, Dr. Shatzer was able to bring to Johns Hopkins expertise in performance-based student assessment and standardized patient technology. This technology, which is well documented in the medical education literature,[2] provides faculty and students with a readily available patient population for the teaching and testing of student skills. Because all students work up the same patient cases, consistent learning experiences and meaningful comparisons between students are possible. For assessment purposes, evaluation instruments using standardized patients and performance standards associated with these instruments can be developed through faculty consensus, permitting fairer and more objective assessments of clinical skills than are possible with traditional methods. Further, when students work up standardized patients, they are required to do so without help from other health professionals. As a result, the quality of their performance reflects their individual knowledge and skills. Standardized patients and their use in performance-based assessments thus produce a better, more controlled, and more thorough measure of clinical competence than is possible with other available methods of teaching and assessment.

To optimize this technology, the Clinical Education Center is well equipped with audiovisual and medical equipment. Students can interact with a standardized patient in this facility as they would with a real patient in an outpatient setting. A stationary video camera and an omnidirectional microphone are strategically mounted to capture the most important aspects of each student-patient encounter. Taping of the encounters is performed by a recorder remotely located in the video monitor room, which also contains a small monitor for each exam room, so that faculty can observe encounters or review tapes at a later date. Tapes are also a powerful tool for providing feedback to students regarding their performance and for providing the Clinical Education Center with quality checks of standardized patient performances. The center consists of nine fully equipped examination rooms, a conference room (which is also wired for audiovisual output), a central monitoring room, staff offices, and storage.

A workshop was held in June 1994 to demonstrate the uses of standardized patient technology for Johns Hopkins faculty and for selected faculty from the Baltimore/Washington Consortium of Medical Schools. Approximately forty faculty attended the workshop, which was conducted by invited leaders in the field of standardized patients. Four areas were addressed: (1) teaching with standardized patients; (2) end-of-clerkship testing; (3) high-stakes testing (for promotion and graduation); and (4) score interpretation and standard setting. Participants acquired hands-on experience working with standardized patients and discussed issues related to their use, validity, and reliability. The workshop helped solidify interest in using standardized patients among the faculty of the six schools. Several subsequent projects for the Clinical Education Center can be traced to this introductory workshop.

The Clinical Education Center staff consists of a head trainer, who is responsible for the overall quality of training and oversees the day-to-day activities of the center, including recruitment of standardized patients, project estimates, and scheduling.

At Johns Hopkins, end-of-clerkship exams and teaching with standardized patients have become a stable if small, part of the new curriculum. The Obstetrics and Gynecology Clerkship and the new Ambulatory Clerkship in Internal Medicine both use standardized patient technology in performance-based final examinations to assess basic clinical skills. Both also have benefited from this method as a means to assess curriculum issues and teaching focus. However, the fact that direct costs for standardized patients are charged to departments is a budgetary concern for some departments. The Psychiatry Clerkship faculty, for example, enthusiastically embrace a performance examination for clerkship students but cannot obtain funding for it from the department.

Standardized patients are used in the second-year Physician and Society course to teach students how to interact with patients who react emotionally to illness. In small groups, students take turns interviewing a patient who, in the course of the encounter, displays various normal emotional reactions to illness (in this case, a husband's illness). These include anger, sadness, and guilt. The encounters provide students with an opportunity to practice some basic communication skills and to become aware of their own reactions to patients who express these common emotions.

The Clinical Education Center is used for other instructional purposes as well. A major consumer of the center's time and space is the second-year Clinical Skills course, which teaches basic skills in history taking and the physical examination. Here students conduct examinations on each other and use the rooms for small-group discussions regarding patients who have been evaluated by them in the hospital. Various departments use the conference room for student seminars and case presentations.

Assessing Student Clinical Skills

The strategic location of the Clinical Education Center in the Baltimore-Washington area, where a broad base of students is available, has enabled the center to become a research site for the National Board of Medical Examiners and the

Educational Commission for Foreign Medical Graduates in their study of performance-based testing for licensure. As a result, the center has secured projects with these organizations for the past three years. These projects have served several purposes. They have helped these organizations further their research on the feasibility, validity, and reliability of performance-based examinations as part of their licensing and certification process. The projects have also served to introduce faculty from area schools to the requirements and benefits of high-stakes testing with standardized patients. For example, these faculty have been introduced to case development issues, training and exam implementation requirements, and methods for scoring and standards setting associated with performance-based tests that use standardized patients. The involvement of faculty in these activities strengthens the dissemination of the standardized patient method as an innovation in curricular change. This, in turn, has allowed the center to grow and stabilize as the dissemination of this new technology spreads to other health care training applications.

Clinical Staff Development

In addition to helping students to learn and be fairly assessed, standardized patients give clinical staff the opportunity to practice, or be assessed for, difficult communication skills. In a standardized environment, trainees can refine and enhance skills to an extent that is otherwise difficult or impossible to attain.

The Clinical Education Center staff have actively sought standardized patient projects that address challenging communication issues because these challenges present particularly difficult training demands in real encounters with patients and families. Projects have focused on emotion-laden settings where physicians are faced with communicating bad news or counseling a family on end-of-life decisions. For example, the Clinical Education Center runs a one-day workshop in which pediatric residents learn to effectively communicate bad news to parents. Standardized parents are trained to provide realistic encounters for the residents and feedback regarding their performance.

In a related project, the Department of Neurology's intensive care unit and the Johns Hopkins Hospital Ethics Committee will collaborate to develop a training and assessment model for improving end-of-life communication and counseling skills. Included in this model are standardized encounters with family or patients to assist in the training of unit personnel. The participants, who will include house staff, faculty, and nursing staff, will be able to work alone or as team members.

The Clinical Education Center is involved in another research project with the Department of Pediatrics to assess pediatric residents in telephone management skills. Individuals will be trained to portray parents who telephone the physician for medical advice. Standardization will enable the investigators to assess all residents on the basis of the same communication variables and to determine which skills most influence patient satisfaction and compliance.

We believe that projects such as these from the Clinical Education Center will enhance the overall quality of clinical instruction and health care training at Johns Hopkins. During its next five years, the center will move to establish a secure place in the milieu of the academic center and to become a recognized leader of innovative educational development and research throughout the medical education community.

Notes

1. A. H. Goroll and G. Morrison, *Core medicine clerkship curriculum guide* (Washington, D.C.: Society of General Internal Medicine, 1995).

2. C. van der Vlueten and D. B. Swanson, "Assessment of clinical skills with standardized patients: State of the art," *Teaching and Learning in Medicine* 2 (1990): 58–76; D. G. Kassebaum and M. B. Anderson, eds., "Proceedings of the AAMC's Consensus Conference on the Use of Standardized Patients in the Teaching and Evaluation of Clinical Skills," *Academic Medicine* 68 (1993): 437–83; and T. A. Mast and M. B. Anderson, eds., "Annex to the proceedings of the AAMC's Consensus Conference on the Use of Standardized Patients in the Teaching and Evaluation of Clinical Skills," *Teaching and Learning in Medicine* 6 (1994): 2–67.

9

Evaluation of the Curriculum

John H. Shatzer, Ph.D., Lucy A. Mead, Sc.M.,
Victor Velculescu, K. Joseph Hurt,
and Michael J. Klag, M.D.

Program evaluation in medical schools provides an organized way to assure faculty, students, the school administration, and the general public that medical education is of high quality. Evaluation primarily determines whether concordance exists between the intended goals of a school's medical curriculum and selected important outcomes. A program evaluation plan also addresses process-related issues, such as whether the content of the curriculum is embraced by faculty and students, teaching methods are deemed appropriate, the learning environment is supportive, and assessment procedures are valid.[1] In monitoring a new curriculum, the task of program evaluation is to assess the current educational practice and outcomes and to measure them against the outcomes that occur as a result of the revision process.

External Evaluation by the Robert Wood Johnson Foundation

The Robert Wood Johnson Foundation (RWJF), which provided planning and implementation grants for our new curriculum, employed an external evaluation team to assess the foundation's program of grants to eight medical schools. In its evaluation of the new curricula at individual schools, including Johns Hopkins, the team sought to answer the following broad questions:

1. How did each school change its basic science curriculum?
2. How did each school modify its clinical curriculum?
3. How has the governing structure of each school been modified to facilitate educational change?
4. What is the interaction between the values and culture of the institution and the dynamics of the change process and its consequences?

5. Which of the above changes can be persuasively attributed to the efforts of RWJF rather than to more general trends in medical education?
6. What impact have (selected) elements of the initiatives had on the general reform in medical education in the United States?
7. What are the common opportunities for and roadblocks to fundamental reform in education in U.S. medical schools, and what has been learned in this program about how to influence them positively?[2]

This external evaluation plan concentrated on the role of Johns Hopkins in the process of change at the national level rather than on the more specific school/student outcomes that were the result of the Johns Hopkins initiative. Measurement sources for the RWJF's external evaluation included faculty surveys and onsite interviews with deans, program leaders, students, and faculty. The presence of this external evaluation plan permitted each of the medical schools that was studied to focus its internal evaluation on other aspects of change valued by the school itself.

Johns Hopkins Internal Evaluation

The new curriculum plan specified seven broad initiatives (listed in chapter 2) to improve the educational process for Johns Hopkins medical students. Consistent with the planned curricular revision and the general goals of an evaluation plan, the school of medicine developed a model to guide the evaluation of the implementation and outcomes of the seven initiatives. This model is based on the work of Spooner et al.,[3] which outlines the practical aspects of curriculum evaluation: the why, what, and how of evaluating an educational program, its participants, and the process by which the program operates. The remainder of this chapter describes the internal evaluation process at Johns Hopkins, as shown in figure 9.1. The process reflects the goals of our initiative and the mission and culture of the institution, and is bound by imposed logistical and fiscal realities as well as by the inherent measurement limitations of the model.

Why Evaluate?

Our first task was to agree on why it was desirable and important to evaluate the curriculum revision at Johns Hopkins. It had been a long time since a major revision was undertaken, and faculty, quite reasonably, asked how the revision would better prepare medical school graduates to be practicing physicians. The initiatives represented a major commitment of faculty time and resources, and it was necessary to justify that commitment in our early discussions of revision

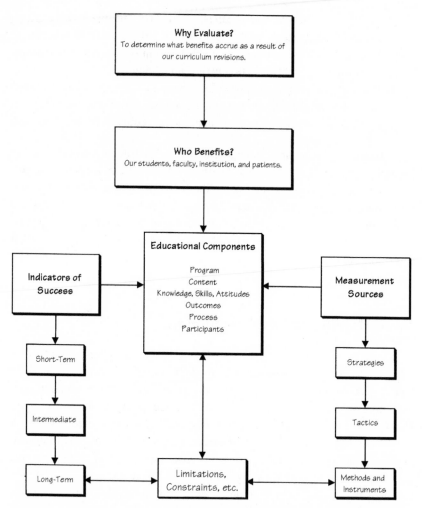

Figure 9.1   Model for curriculum evaluation at Johns Hopkins School of Medicine. Adapted, by permission, from B. Jolly and M. MacDonald, figure 1, in *Essays on curriculum development and formulation in medicine,* ed. G. Page (report of the Second Cambridge Conference, University of Brititsh Columbia, 1989), p. 124.

proposals. In response to this general concern, we designed our evaluation to determine what benefits would accrue as a result of curriculum revisions.

Who Benefits?

Our evaluation plan had to document who would benefit from the curriculum revision and evaluation. The most important beneficiaries would be our students, who must be well educated and trained to begin their practice of medicine, but others should also benefit from this innovation process. Faculty should acquire new teaching techniques and opportunities to disseminate their ideas through educational research and presentations at other institutions or at conferences. Their teaching efforts should be valued more highly by the institution, as evidenced by revisions in the criteria for promotion and tenure. The school should benefit from being viewed by the public as responsive to the changing medical care environment and as a creator of educational innovation. The new curriculum and evaluation might also influence the kind of students who apply to the school of medicine. Finally, patients should become the ultimate beneficiaries of the curriculum revision, as reflected in our graduates' desire for lifelong learning and a resultant sustained excellence in the quality of care.

Educational Components

For purposes of evaluation, we have categorized our indicators of success under three educational components—the program, the process, and the participants—and have compared these components in the old and new curricula. The educational *program*, for example, is evaluated in terms of content and outcomes under the two curricula; the educational *process* is evaluated in terms of student and faculty views about it; and the educational *participants*—students and faculty—are studied on various dimensions, such as student learning styles, student views of the learning environment, the faculty's initiative in the use of innovative instructional designs, and faculty rewards for the implementation of such designs.

Thinking in terms of these components helped us to define the indicators of success that would be used in our evaluation plan. The indicators then needed to be matched with sources of measurement that would provide clear evidence for the success or failure of our efforts. Not all indicators can be matched to measurement sources; for example, the indicator "practice better medicine" expresses a laudable goal for any medical curriculum, but to achieve agreement on appropriate or feasible methods of measuring it is difficult. Our measurement sources had to be both feasible and accessible to us through valid instruments.

Indicators of Success

In defining the indicators of success for the new curriculum, we used aspects of student outcomes and process variables that increasingly have been recognized as important in medical school curricula[4] and also have been consistently valued by Johns Hopkins students in their evaluations of the curriculum. For example, our students have indicated consistently over the past several years that the density of the first-year basic science curriculum made it difficult to fully appreciate the vital relationships between the basic sciences and the practice of medicine. In addition, the first-year curriculum allowed little time for personal or professional pursuits such as community volunteer work or individual research projects. Evaluating the success of our new basic science curriculum would mean, in part, evaluating the impact of the reduced density of didactic instruction on students' use of time and their opportunity to pursue outside interests. In annual exit evaluations conducted by the Association of American Medical Colleges (AAMC) for graduating medical students, our students also consistently reported concerns over the lack of outpatient learning opportunities. As a result of our initiative to establish increased outpatient teaching experiences, we expected this perception to change.

Our design incorporated indicators of short-term, intermediate, and long-term outcomes in order to measure success as students and faculty progressed through their career paths. By assessing short-term outcomes (such as confirmation that changes in teaching have altered students' view of their learning environment) we would capture the information needed to make corrections as we introduced further curricular changes. By assessing intermediate outcomes (such as students' performance on examinations or the effects of the new curriculum on their choice of career specialties) we would detect trends in students' perception of their experiences and determine how the new curricular emphases might contribute to lasting performance effects. Finally, by assessing long-term outcomes (such as career satisfaction among our practicing physicians, their approaches to patient care, and their humanistic abilities) we would document enduring changes produced, at least in part, by the new curriculum.

While outcome evaluations typically focus on student performance measures, such as grade point average, we chose to focus on other student variables for two reasons. First, there is no satisfactory single gold standard for student performance. Second, no objective performance measures were available to us from the years before the curriculum change for purposes of comparison. Grade point averages were not likely to be comparable, given that assessment methods differed under the old and new curricula.

One outcome measure that medical schools frequently choose in assessing curricular changes is United States Medical Licensing Examination (USMLE) scores. These are appealing to faculty because the examinations are a respected, externally developed competency measure that provides a school with a national calibration of student achievement and, thus, of curricular success. At Johns Hopkins, however, students never were required by the school to pass the National Board of Medical Examiners' Part I and II examinations for promotion or graduation. Most Hopkins students did not participate in the NBME examinations, but elected instead to participate in the FLEX examination during their internships to meet their licensure requirements. Consequently, student data on NBME Part I and II examinations are sparse. The potential usefulness of NBME data in an evaluation of the revised curriculum was further complicated by the implementation of the new USMLE Step Examinations in 1992 as a single path to licensure. All U.S. students are now required to take these newly designed examinations. As a result, we decided to use USLME scores to help assess future trends in student and curricular success under the new curriculum.

Finally, we felt that new curricular approaches with new goals warranted new assessment methods. Therefore, while we decided to continue monitoring student performance outcomes through traditional objective indicators, we believed that other indicators would be equally important over the long term.

Measurement Sources

Because traditional measurement sources other than the USMLE either were unavailable to us or were not chosen as valued indicators, we reviewed the literature on medical education and contacted medical educators at institutions that had incorporated new curricula. Through these sources of information we identified existing evaluation tools that addressed our interests and chosen indicators. We selected three short-term instruments designed to assess the aspects of the students' school environment and approaches to learning that we anticipated would change. These instruments are described in a later section ("Evaluation of the New Curriculum"). We also developed a questionnaire of our own to assess first-year students' use of unscheduled class time in the afternoons and their views on that aspect of the new curriculum. The issue of unscheduled time was of interest to the faculty and the school administration because, under the new basic science curriculum, faculty had agreed to restrict lectures to two hours per day on average and to finish all didactic teaching by 1 P.M.

Other aspects of our evaluation plan address specific components of the new curriculum and attempt to answer content-based questions of curricular success. In the Physician and Society course, for example, evaluation questionnaires frequently were distributed to students to assess their experience of this new course, and focus groups also were held to gather detailed student comments and suggestions. Early in the curricular revision process, focus group evaluations were conducted after every unit in the Physician and Society course to guarantee feedback to course leaders regarding the quality of learning and instruction. As adjustments were made in the course and refinements were developed that addressed critical student issues, these evaluations were conducted at longer intervals. This change was consistent with the overall plan for maintenance evaluation in the course.

Table 9.1 presents a matrix of the indicators of success and the measurement

Table 9.1 Jhu-Som Indicators of Successful Curricular Reform

Indicators of Success	Medical School Years	Graduate/ Professional Years	Measurement Sources
Student Outcomes			a = School-based assessments
Satisfaction with the curriculum	b, c, p, q	h, s	b = Standardized questionnaires
Use of free time	b, e, o	h	c = Focus group sessions
Use of life-long learning skills	f, i, j	h, s	d = Curriculum syllabi/documents
Increase in outpatient experiences	d, l, p, s	c, h	e = NBME Step Examinations
Use of medical informatics knowledge and skills	a, b, c, i, n	c, h, n	f = School performance-based exams
Use of effective patient communication skills	d, f, o	s	g = Residency focus groups
Understanding of evidence-based medicine	a, d, f, i,o	e, s	h = Post-graduate questionnaires
Choice of career pathways	b, c, o, p	g, h, s	i = Computer-based software use audits
Understanding of cost-effective medicine	a, d, f, i, m, o	e, s	j = Library medline audits

Understanding of basic science principles/mechanisms	a, d, f, i, m, o	a, d, f, i, k, m, o
Understanding of disease processes/mechanisms	a, d, f, i, m, o	e, s
Effective and appropriate use of physician tools	a, d, f, i, k, m, o	e, s
Application of ethical principles to patient care	a, d, f, i, k, m, o	e, s

Faculty Development

Understanding/use of new teaching methods	d, f, l, r, s, t, q, k, u
Understanding/use of new methods of assessment	a, f, l, q, t
Understanding of methods/uses of program evaluation	c, s, t
Openness to new educational ideas	d, e, q
Pursuit of answers to educational problems	l, q, r, t
Participation in faculty development	r, u

k = Observations of small group learning

l = Course evaluations by students

m = NBME shelf examinations

n = Needs assessments

o = Academic record

p = AAMC exit surveys

q = Student Curriculum Committee surveys

r = Faculty interviews and questionnaires

s = Program directors questionnaires

t = Publications, presentations

u = Institutional surveys, statistics

Source: Adopted from the University of Kentucky School of Medicine, Office of Education.

217

sources that we have used or plan to use, together with those that are available to us should we decide to use them. The remainder of this chapter describes our current methods of collecting data and some proposed evaluation variables. We plan to submit additional information for publication or public presentation as we complete each evaluation component, or as we accumulate and analyze data that may be of interest to people in the field of medical education.

Assessment of the Traditional Curriculum

Few historical data are available on former Johns Hopkins students, particularly standardized outcome data that might be compared with current student outcomes under the new curriculum. This lack of data is compounded by the lack of a continuous systematic evaluation plan at Johns Hopkins prior to the initiation of the new curriculum. (There was, however, substantial interest in curriculum reform evaluation among both faculty and students.)

Students' View of the Traditional Curriculum

Formal student input into the evaluation plan occurred early in the Robert Wood Johnson Foundation curriculum initiative and provided curriculum planners with additional information for the reform process. The results of student-run surveys also underscored many of the concerns identified by faculty regarding the traditional educational program and individual courses. One of these surveys assessed students' views of the old curriculum. A second evaluated students' reactions to the first iteration of the redesigned basic science year in order to provide curriculum planners with additional information regarding possible further refinements. Both initiatives were managed by students with support from faculty and the dean's office.

The first student survey originated from discussions in the Educational Policy Committee (EPC) when plans for the new curriculum were being considered.[5] Third-year student representatives on the committee expressed interest in performing an evaluation of the current, traditional first-year curriculum. The students and the director of medical education services planned a series of student focus groups. These groups were comprised mostly of students in their second year of medical school but also included third- and fourth-year students. Each group met to develop issues related to the basic science curriculum. Chairpersons from each focus group then met to develop consensus issues to report to the faculty.

The student EPC representatives met with appropriate faculty leaders to discuss the findings and recommendations. The focus groups had offered comments that were course-specific, for the most part, but that confirmed the desirability of changes that faculty had proposed on a broader scale. Among the most important shared priorities were (1) better integration of the basic sciences with the clinical experiences (faculty and students suggested similar means for introducing skill- and attitude-based learning into the first-year curriculum); (2) coordination of course material across departments, to be achieved through a modular or block-type calendar system; and (3) interactive and active learning, to be encouraged through a reduction of lectures, an increase in small-group instruction, and the scheduling of more free time for independent learning. To complete the evaluation process, a faculty response to the report was summarized for participating students.

Student focus groups were also organized to evaluate the current, traditional second-year and clinical curricula.[6] For the clinical years, the focus groups highlighted four needs: (1) increased ambulatory and primary care experience; (2) standardization of teaching and clinical experiences; (3) more comprehensive and multidisciplinary advising; and (4) flexibility in scheduling. Needs highlighted for the second-year curriculum included (1) better integration of the basic science courses with the clinical sciences; (2) greater coordination of course materials across departments; and (3) active and interactive learning, for example, in case-based and computer-based modalities.

Both focus-group projects provided the curriculum coordinators with valuable student evaluations of the current educational programs and added an important validation process to the design of the new curriculum. The reports that came out of these projects, along with a growing body of national data about medical education in the United States, as evidenced by the General Professional Education of the Physician (GPEP) and ACME-TRI reports,[7] served as our school's benchmark for change.

Evaluation of the New Curriculum

Measurement Sources

The evaluation of the new curriculum began in 1992 after the first iteration of the new first-year basic science curriculum. Three standardized instruments were chosen to assess student changes by comparing selected variables under the old and new curricula and in successive iterations of the new curriculum. These instruments, chosen for the purpose of evaluating short-term and intermediate student goals, were the Medical Student Learning Environment Survey, the Learning Preference Inventory, and the Cognitive Behavior Survey.[8] The Learning Preference Inventory, designed to assess students' individual learning styles from self-report, was abandoned after the first year in lieu of the Cognitive Behavior Survey. (We decided that the Learning Reference Inventory did not reflect current knowledge in psychology and education; moreover, students regarded it as less credible than other questionnaires, leaving doubt about the validity of their responses.) In addition, we developed another questionnaire to assess students' use of the increased free time available under the new curriculum.

The evaluation plan also included selected prematriculation and other medical school outcome variables. The prematriculation variables were collected to help us determine whether various factors, such as undergraduate major, were associated with acceptance of curricular change and how they affected student performance and attitudes. Other outcome and process data that were included in the evaluation plan, such as USMLE scores and course evaluations, are being collected in an effort to monitor continuously the effects of the curricular revisions and to provide an ongoing source of feedback to course directors and curriculum coordinators.

Beginning with the 1992/93 school year, all students were asked to complete three instruments after finishing their basic science year: the Medical Student Learning Environment Survey (to assess students' views on the learning environment under the old and new curricula), the Cognitive Behavior Survey (to assess student perceptions of their individual approaches to learning), and the free-time questionnaire (to assess students' use of free time under the new first-year curriculum). First-year students were asked to complete the three questionnaires in a single sitting, resulting in a participation/return rate of about 70 percent. Second-year students were mailed their questionnaires, resulting in a return rate of about 60 percent. The preliminary results are reported below. Also reported are the results of the student-run survey to assess the new curriculum and the faculty's assessment of student performance in the new curriculum.

Medical Student Learning Environment Survey

The Medical Student Learning Environment Survey assesses six dimensions of students' view of their learning environment during their first two years of medical school. It consists of six subscales, which measure students' perceptions of (1) openness (the degree to which the educational environment allows for interests other than medicine); (2) nurturance (supportiveness of faculty); (3) meaningful experience (the meaningfulness of students' learning experiences in relation to problems they will encounter as physicians); (4) student interaction

Table 9.2 Distribution of Learning Environment Survey Scores
(First-Year Students Under New Curriculum, Classes of 1996–98)

Subscale	Number of Items	N	Possible Subscale Range (Midpoint)	Mean	SD
Openness	5	241	4–20 (12)	13.3	2.8
Nurturance	4	241	4–16 (10)	13.2	1.8
Meaningful experience	6	239	4–24 (14)	16.9	2.8
Student interaction	5	238	4–20 (12)	15.2	2.6
Emotional climate	9	234	4–36 (20)	25.1	4.8
Flexibility	4	239	4–16 (10)	11.5	1.9

(closeness between students); (5) emotional climate (general atmosphere of supportiveness); and (6) flexibility (degree of flexibility or rigidity of the learning environment). For each item on the survey, students respond to a four-point Likert-type scale (4 = this happens very frequently; 3 = this happens fairly regularly; 2 = this happens once in a while; 1 = this rarely happens). A number of items are scored negatively; the resulting score in a given subscale is the sum of the signed values of the Likert scores. Higher scores reflect more favorable student perceptions of their learning environment. Tables 9.2 and 9.3 show the distribution of scores. Because first-year scores were the same for the first three classes that participated in the revised curriculum, the results provided in table 9.2 are for the first three classes combined.

Table 9.3 shows the scores of two groups of second-year students on the Learning Environment Survey, representing the class of 1995 and the class of 1996, respectively. The class of 1995 was the last class to complete its second year under the old curriculum; the class of 1996 was the first class to complete its second year under the new curriculum. The scores for openness, nurturance, student interaction, and emotional climate did not differ significantly under the old and new curricula, although the nurturance and student interaction scores rose slightly. The scores for meaningful experience and flexibility were significantly higher under the new curriculum. The scores that rose under the new curriculum reflect values that were consciously incorporated into its design.

As a next step, we sought to determine whether there was a correlation between students' perception of the learning environment and their academic success, as reflected by grade point average. Table 9.4 shows the results. First-year grade point average was positively associated with students' perception that the openness of the curriculum allowed for outside interests ($p < .001$). It was also positively associated with the perception of the learning experience as mean-

Table 9.3 Distribution of Learning Environment Survey Scores (Second-Year Students under Old and New Curricula, Classes of 1995 and 1996, Respectively)

Subscale	N	Mean	SD
Openness			
Old curriculum	65	10.8	2.7
New curriculum	77	10.0	2.9
Nurturance			
Old curriculum	65	11.6	1.8
New curriculum	77	12.2	1.9
Meaningful experience[a]			
Old curriculum	65	14.0	3.0
New curriculum	77	15.7	3.2
Student interaction			
Old curriculum	65	13.8	2.9
New curriculum	77	14.4	2.6
Emotional climate			
Old curriculum	64	22.0	5.3
New curriculum	77	21.9	4.7
Flexibility[b]			
Old curriculum	64	9.1	1.8
New curriculum	75	10.5	1.9

[a]$p < .05$
[b]$p < .0001$

Table 9.4 Correlation (r) of First-Year Students' Learning Environment Survey Scores with First-Year Grade Point Average (Classes of 1996–98)

Subscale	r, First-Year GPA ($N = 197$)
Openness	0.24[a]
Nurturance	0.11
Meaningful experience	0.23[b]
Student interaction	0.08
Emotional climate	0.24[a]
Flexibility	0.12

[a]$p < .001$
[b]$p < .01$

Table 9.5   Correlations (*r*) of Second-Year Students'
Grade Point Average with Second-Year Learning
Environment Survey Scores
(Class of 1996)

Subscale	r, Second-Year Score ($N = 70$)
Openness	0.11
Nurturance	0.14
Meaningful experience	0.14
Student interaction	0.16
Emotional climate	0.26[a]
Flexibility	0.02

[a]$p < .05$

ingful in relation to problems students would encounter as physicians ($p < .01$). Finally, it was significantly related to students' view of the emotional climate of the first-year curriculum ($p < .001$).

Between students' first and second years of medical school, average scores fell significantly for all of the subscales of the Learning Environment Survey (data not shown). To investigate whether second-year grade point average was associated either with second-year Learning Environment Survey scores or with positive or negative *change* in the scores between a student's first and second years, we examined the scores of the class of 1996, which had completed the Learning Environment Survey in both its first and second years. As shown in table 9.5, the perception of a more supportive emotional climate at the end of the second year was associated with higher grades. Correlation coefficients for the other subscales were also positive but not statistically significant. The associations between grade point average and change in Learning Environment Survey scores were of smaller magnitude, and none were statistically significant.

Cognitive Behavior Survey

The Cognitive Behavior Survey assesses various aspects of student learning and consists of four subscales that measure conceptualization, reflection, memorization, and positive learning experience. The instrument includes Likert-scale questions, fill-in questions, rank-order questions, and open-ended questions, all designed to examine a student's *learning behavior, learning experience,* and *epistemological beliefs.* The Learning Behavior component examines (1) the student's general cognitive processes, that is, the extent to which the student relies on memorization, conceptualization, active construction of a knowledge base, and reflection on what is learned; (2) the student's cognitive representations of knowledge, that is, the extent to which the student uses memorization, visual representations, or explanatory models for learning and remembering; (3) the student's approaches to studying, such as note taking, review of sources, and peer-group study; and (4) the student's perception of the amount of material learned. The Learning Experience component examines student perceptions of the characteristics and quality of the learning experiences. Finally, the Epistemological Beliefs component examines student views on (1) the nature of knowledge; (2) the nature of knowledge acquisition; and (3) the factors the student believes determine his or her level of understanding.

For purposes of this chapter, we report results from the subscales of the Learning Behavior component (conceptualization, reflection, and memorization) and of the Learning Experience component (positive learning experience). Students responded to a seven-point Likert scale (with varying descriptive anchors) for all items in the four subscales. On all subscales a higher score indicates that the behavior or experience is more pronounced. Multiple versions of the Cognitive Behavior Survey address various levels of training in medical school. We chose to use two versions: one that assesses students' learning behavior, learning experience, and epistemological beliefs at their matriculation into medical school, and one that assesses these components when students are about to enter their third-year clinical rotations. The distribution of scores on the Cognitive Behavior Survey for first-year students in the first three classes to participate in the new curriculum is shown in table 9.6. The possible range and calculated midpoint for each subscale are also shown in the table to provide a frame of reference for the score results. For these students, only the conceptualization and positive learning experience scores were substantially higher than the midpoints of their respective subscales; the other two scores were at or near midpoint. Student results in the conceptualization scale, in particular, suggest that

Table 9.6 Distribution of Cognitive Behavior Survey Scores
(First-Year Students under New Curriculum, Classes of 1996–98)

Subscale	Possible Subscale Range	Subscale Midpoint	N	Mean	SD
Conceptualization	12–84	48	286	64.6	8.3
Reflection	6–42	24	291	26.7	5.5
Memorization	11–77	44	284	43.0	10.7
Positive learning experience	9–63	36	289	47.2	8.3

Table 9.7   Distribution of Cognitive Behavior Survey Scores (Second-Year Students under Old and New Curricula, Classes of 1995 and 1996, Respectively)

Subscale	N	Mean	SD
Conceptualization			
Old curriculum	70	59.5[a]	10.7
New curriculum	81	63.0	8.5
Reflection			
Old curriculum	70	25.8	5.4
New curriculum	81	26.0	4.8
Memorization			
Old curriculum	69	47.4	11.1
New curriculum	78	49.9	11.1
Positive learning experience			
Old curriculum	70	40.0[a]	8.5
New curriculum	81	42.6	7.7

[a] $p < .05$

many important elements of learning for understanding were incorporated into the new curriculum.

Table 9.7 compares the Cognitive Behavior Survey scores of second-year students under the new curriculum (class of 1996) with those of second-year students under the old curriculum (class of 1995). Two subscales, conceptualization and positive learning experience, received significantly different scores under the old and new curricula. As in table 9.6, the direction of the associations is consistent with the intended goals of the new curriculum. As is shown in table 9.8, no significant correlations were found between the subscale scores and grade-

Table 9.8   Correlation (r) of Second-Year Students' Cognitive Behavior Survey Scores with Second-Year Grade Point Average (Class of 1996)

Subscale	r, Second-Year GPA
Conceptualization	0.00
Reflection	−0.17
Memorization	0.12
Positive learning experience	0.13

point average for second-year students. This finding suggests that there is an incongruency between the value that students under the new curriculum place on strategies for learning and the way that they are evaluated to determine grade point average. If the second-year evaluation system is left unchanged, this could influence students' approaches to learning despite curriculum revisions.

Free-Time Survey

An instrument was constructed specifically to address the issue of the use of unscheduled time by first-year students. Before the schoolwide curricular revisions, the first year included approximately 20 hours of lectures per week. Under the new curriculum, first-year faculty agreed to present no more than 2 hours of lectures each day. Despite the addition of new small-group components and a clinical experience, the overall decrease in lecture time provided students with an average of 9–12 free hours per week that traditionally had been spent in class. The questionnaire addressed three main questions regarding this increased free time. The data from two surveys collected from first-year students (classes of 1996 and 1997) were combined for all analyses ($N = 193$).

1. What activities did students value most during their unscheduled time?

Students were asked to rate the value of five major free-time categories on a scale of 1 to 6 (1 = most important; 6 = least important). The categories were (a) preparation or review of course materials; (b) independent study of additional materials related to courses; (c) career-related activities apart from coursework; (d) personal time (e.g., time spent with family and friends); and (e) health maintenance. A sixth option permitted students to write in other valued activities.

Thirty-six percent of the students ranked preparation or review of course materials first during weekday afternoons; 36 percent ranked personal time first. Health-maintenance activities and career-related activities were ranked first by 14 and 10 percent of the students, respectively.

2. How did students use their free time?

For each day of the week, students circled their free-time activities (selected from the six categories listed under question 1) in a typical week during the academic year. Each weekday was divided into afternoon and evening blocks. Saturdays and Sundays were listed as a composite weekend category of afternoon and evening time. Students were instructed to list no more than two activities during each time block.

Table 9.9 shows the distribution of self-reported student activities during un-

Table 9.9 Distribution of Free-Time Activities on Weekday Afternoons
under New Curriculum
(First-Year Students, Classes of 1996 and 1997) (*N* = 193)

Activity	Number of Weekday Afternoons	
	Mean	SD
Preparation or review of course materials	4.9	2.8
Independent study	0.9	1.8
Career-related activities	1.2	1.6
Personal time	3.2	2.2
Health maintenance	2.6	2.6
Other	0.6	1.4

scheduled weekday afternoons in the new curriculum. (We report only weekday afternoon activities because this time block concerned faculty the most.) Students devoted the most time to the preparation or review of course materials; personal time came second. Their use of weekday afternoons for other listed activities varied widely, suggesting that students used this time in accordance with their own needs and values. Thus, the increase in unscheduled time allowed students greater flexibility in determining how best to approach the demands of their schooling.

3. Did students feel that the amount of unscheduled time was appropriate?

This question was assessed by asking whether the unscheduled time afforded the student during the year was about the right amount. Students responded by indicating that there was too little, about the right amount, or too much free time.

Eighty-eight percent of the students thought that the amount of unscheduled time was about right. Only 7 percent thought that the amount of free time was excessive; 5 percent reported that there was still too little free time.

Selected prematriculation and medical school outcome variables also will be included in the free-time component of the future overall analysis of program success. Prematriculation variables will be chosen to help determine whether factors such as undergraduate major are associated with students' use of free time. It is possible, for example, that students who have a nonscience undergraduate degree spend more time studying curriculum-related materials than do students who are better acquainted with the scientific concepts addressed in medical school. Conversely, students with nonscience undergraduate degrees may use more free time for volunteer projects than do typical pre-med majors. M.D.-Ph.D. students may spend more of their unscheduled time on research projects than do regular M.D. students. Students who enter Johns Hopkins with a graduate science degree (usually this is a Ph.D.) might be expected to spend less time on the curriculum, choosing instead to pursue other professional or personal interests.

Student Evaluation of the New Curriculum

Students played a major role in evaluating the new first-year curriculum when it was first implemented, using both qualitative and quantitative methods.[9] To evaluate their experience, in 1992 students created the Student Curriculum Committee (SCC), a representative body designed to offer concurrent and retrospective analyses of first-year coursework.

The SCC was composed of student representatives from eight small-group sections, each of which elected one representative and one alternate at the start of each school year. The representatives collected curriculum assessments from their groups every week and met at least twice monthly to discuss and analyze curricular issues. The SCC met with first-year course directors during and after each course and with all first-year course instructors at the end of the year. It presented summaries of student analyses of the curriculum and offered specific suggestions for the presentation, content, and structure of individual courses and for methods of student testing and evaluation.

To quantitate individuals' sentiments on the new curriculum, the SCC conducted anonymous student and faculty surveys in May 1993 and June 1994. The surveys were entitled First-Year New Curriculum I (FYNC1) and First-Year New Curriculum II (FYNC2), respectively; each included student and faculty questionnaires. The student questionnaire asked for students' overall impressions of the first-year curriculum and their assessment of specific curricular components, study resources, grading systems, and examination types. The faculty questionnaire asked for faculty's impressions of the first-year curriculum and of student qualities. Survey questions were scaled from 1 (low) to 5 (high), with 3 as the neutral response. The FYNC1 survey (conducted in 1993) asked faculty members to compare their students under the new curriculum with students under the previous curriculum. In the FYNC2 survey (conducted in 1994), faculty members rated the new curriculum on the basis of their general experience.

Student Response to SCC Surveys

The completed student questionnaires provided an overall analysis of student satisfaction with the various components of the first-year curriculum. A high pro-

Table 9.10   Students' Mean Ratings of General Impressions, Curriculum Components, and Study Resources in the First-Year New Curriculum, 1992/93 (FYNC1) and 1993/94 (FYNC2)

Items Rated	FYNC1 (1992/93) $N = 101$		FYNC2 (1993/94) $N = 101$		
	Mean	SD	Mean	SD	p
General Impressions					
First-year new curriculum	4.21	0.71	4.06	0.87	ns
Student-faculty interactions	4.09	0.75	4.00	0.86	ns
Schedule	4.19	0.75	3.97	0.70	< 0.05
Curriculum Components					
Lectures	4.02	0.71	4.07	0.75	ns
Small-group discussions	3.99	0.88	4.14	0.89	ns
Laboratories	3.73	0.78	3.99	0.94	< 0.05
Journal clubs	3.22	1.04	3.13	1.19	ns
Clinical correlations	4.13	0.84	4.04	0.91	ns
Physician and Society course	3.97	0.99	3.35	1.05	< 0.01
Community preceptorship	nd	nd	4.22	0.91	—
Study Resources					
Lecture notes	4.78	0.48	4.79	0.53	ns
Assigned texts	3.53	0.91	3.22	1.00	< 0.05
Other texts	2.77	1.21	2.56	1.14	ns
Out-of-class study groups	3.45	1.17	3.50	1.17	ns
Computer-aided instruction	3.58	1.05	3.88	0.99	< 0.05

Note: Results of Student Curriculum Committee surveys of May 1993 and June 1994. Students rated items on a scale from 1 (low) to 5 (high), with 3 = neutral.

portion of students responded to the surveys: 101 of 123 (82%) for FYNC1 and 101 of 120 (84%) for FYNC2. Both groups of students assessed positively the overall first-year curriculum, overall student-faculty interactions, and the schedule; mean scores ranged from 3.97 to 4.21 for these items (table 9.10). Some students wrote that if they had been asked to rate student-faculty interactions separately for each course, they would have assigned higher scores to courses that devoted more time to small-group discussions.

Students from both years rated lectures, small-group discussions, and clinical correlations highly, with mean scores from 3.99 to 4.14. FYNC1 students felt that the laboratory experience was less valuable than did FYNC2 students (3.73 versus 3.99, $p < 0.05$), possibly because some of the laboratories that were perceived as less instructive were modified or removed after the first year. Both FYNC1 and FYNC2 students judged the journal club, a weekly discussion of a journal paper that was related to course content, to be the least valuable component of the curriculum but nevertheless assigned positive mean scores of 3.22 and 3.13, respectively. FYNC1 students rated the Physician and Society course significantly higher than did FYNC2 students (3.97 versus 3.35, $p < 0.01$), possibly because several changes in unit topics were made for the second iteration of the course.

Students in both years gave very high ratings to the detailed lecture notes provided by instructors for each lecture, assigning mean scores of 4.78 and 4.79 (median $= 5$). FYNC1 students rated assigned texts at 3.53, computer-aided instruction at 3.58. FYNC2 students were less enthusiastic about assigned texts (3.22, $p < 0.05$) but more enthusiastic about computer-aided instruction (3.88, $p < 0.05$). The increase in computer-aided instructional software in the second iteration may account for this difference. Out-of-class study groups received mean scores of 3.45 and 3.50 from FYNC1 and FYNC2 students, respectively. However, large standard deviations around the means indicate variability in out-of-class group participation. Additional texts, often recommended by individual instructors, were generally unused.

To identify potential predictors of overall curriculum assessment, the correlation of assessments of individual components of the curriculum with overall assessment of the first year was examined. The components whose assessments correlated most highly with overall assessment of the first year were student-faculty interactions, general schedule, lectures, and clinical correlations. There were no significant negative correlations with students' overall impression of the first-year curriculum.

Faculty Response to SCC Surveys

The faculty questionnaires were distributed to faculty members who regularly taught the first-year curriculum or were instructors in the weekly journal clubs. For the FYNC1 survey, 44 of 60 faculty members (73%) responded; for FYNC2, 53 of 90 (58%) responded. Faculty members rated all student qualities under the new curriculum above the average score of 3 (table 9.11) and gave high scores for students' knowledge, attendance, preparedness, and attentiveness/enthusiasm. These scores showed no significant differences by year. There was a modest rise in perceived student test performance from FYNC1 to FYNC2, possibly due to better coordination of the overall curriculum in the second year.

For both years, faculty also gave high ratings to student-faculty interactions, probably due at least in part to the increased time that students and faculty members spent together in small groups and journal clubs under the new curriculum.

Table 9.11 Faculty's Mean Ratings of General Impressions and Observed Student Qualities in the First-Year New Curriculum, 1992/93 (FYCN1) and 1993/94 (FYNC2)

Items Rated	FYNC1 (1992/93) $N = 44$		FYNC2 (1993/94) $N = 57$		
	Mean	SD	Mean	SD	p
General Impressions					
Student-faculty interactions	4.00	1.04	4.18	0.84	ns
Respondent's enthusiasm	3.93	1.00	nd	nd	—
Observed Student Qualities					
Knowledge	3.63	0.91	3.81	0.69	ns
Test performance	3.25	0.72	3.64	0.73	< 0.05
Attendance	3.69	0.89	3.57	1.12	ns
Preparedness	3.76	0.90	3.58	0.89	ns
Attentivenss/enthusiasm	4.13	0.73	4.01	0.91	ns

Note: Results of Student Curriculum Committee surveys of May 1993 and June 1994. Faculty rated items on a scale from 1 (low) to 5 (high), with 3 = neutral.

FYNC1 faculty members reported feeling more enthusiastic about teaching than in previous years. FYNC2 faculty were not asked about their own level of enthusiasm.

SCC Survey Conclusions

The information collected from students and faculty members in the FYNC1 and FYNC2 surveys indicated that educational reform was received positively at Johns Hopkins. The basis for the reforms—that an improved curriculum would include varied pedagogical approaches and additional perspectives on the science and art of medicine—was perceived favorably. Both FYNC1 and FYNC2 students positively assessed their overall experience, schedule, and interaction with the faculty. FYNC1 and FYNC2 faculty rated students in the new curriculum as highly knowledgeable, prepared, and enthusiastic.

Our survey data and individual discussions with medical students suggested that students preferred a curriculum that incorporated lectures, problem-based small-group discussions, journal clubs, laboratories, and independent learning. The various components of the new curriculum were rated highly by FYNC1 and FYNC2 students. No component received a mean score below 3 (neutral) on our five-point scale, and many of the components showed positive correlations with one another. Although some components may have qualified as predictors of overall satisfaction with the new first-year curriculum, the survey results suggested that nearly all of the new components were valuable to the students. No student respondent asked for increased lecture time or for a more traditional educational format.

The clinical components of the first-year curriculum scored among the highest in the student surveys. Written comments indicated that some students regarded these as the best parts of the new curriculum, that the clinical correlations helped students to remember the basic science of specific diseases, and that seeing patients each week improved student morale.

The student scores on study techniques indicated that students under the new curriculum had identifiable study preferences. Lecture notes prepared by the faculty lecturers, with complete text and diagrams, were assessed very positively; the median score for lecture notes was 5 on our five-point scale. In their written comments, students expressed appreciation for high-quality notes in a standardized format applied consistently from one course or lecture to the next. Likewise, computer-aided instruction and study groups were assessed highly.

Faculty members gave favorable assessments of student qualities under the new curriculum. No quality received a score lower than 3. Many professors, in written and oral comments, noted that students under the new curriculum were more enthusiastic and more knowledgeable than those of previous years. Some professors also mentioned that students asked more questions in lectures and small groups and read more of the required texts and notes.

Whether students' enthusiasm about their education will translate in future years to increased excellence in patient care, professional leadership, or scientific achievement remains to be seen. Both faculty and students reported positive student-faculty interactions, although some faculty members would have appreciated additional time to meet students, especially in nonclassroom settings. The facilitation of mentoring relationships and professional interactions between students and faculty members is a strong component of the new curriculum. Since neither admission policies nor faculty personnel have changed significantly since the adoption of the new curriculum, it seems reasonable to credit the faculty's perceived improvement in student qualities and student-faculty interactions to the curricular reforms.

The SCC represented the first organized attempt by Johns Hopkins medical students to provide systematic feedback to faculty regarding a new curricular effort. Although written course evaluations had been used at Johns Hopkins for many years, this method often suffered from lack of student participation and from significant delays in the incorporation of student suggestions. The regular dialogue between faculty and medical students facilitated by the SCC helped to increase student involvement in the implementation of the new curriculum and increased the pace of curricular change.

Evaluation of Individual Instructional Components

While the evaluation process described in the preceding sections measured indicators of success in the schoolwide change process, faculty began their own efforts to determine the success of their particular instructional components of the new curriculum. Their efforts are not a part of our evaluation design, but they merit mention here. They concentrate on outcome and process variables that offer a unique view of the impact of curricular changes at Johns Hopkins, and the results eventually will provide faculty with answers to their question regarding the usefulness of the curricular reform. Moreover, it is anticipated that faculty will begin to view evaluation of their instructional components as something that deserves continuous attention. There is evidence to suggest that this is already happening.

First-year curriculum leaders continue to solicit feedback from students as they progress through the year. This is accomplished through a series of small-group discussions between selected class representatives and the first-year course directors, including the first-year curriculum coordinator. In addition, the first-year course directors meet on a regular basis to discuss issues of overall concern to the proper implementation of the first-year curriculum. This is also true of the second-year course directors. These faculty are now planning an overall evaluation of their own efforts in the change process. Communication between the first- and second-year faculty is also increasing as gaps in content coverage continue to be identified and addressed. Third-year clinical clerkship directors began meeting in 1997 to address common issues, including scheduling, student performance, documentation of the teaching efforts of clinical faculty, and other concerns.

Long-Term Evaluation

The long-term goal underlying revision of the curriculum is to produce better physicians. ("Long-term," for purposes of this discussion, means at graduation or later.) Evaluating whether this goal has been achieved is difficult for several reasons, some of which also contribute to the difficulty of evaluating short-term goals, as previously discussed. First, reaching agreement on what constitutes a "better physician" is problematic. Second, if a definition is agreed on, it may not be measurable by any existing technique, or by any technique that feasibly can be employed. Third, long-term assessment (which ideally, takes place when the physician has completed residency and fellowship training) is by nature a slow process; its results are not known until years after the curriculum has been revised and may not be available to guide subsequent phases of the revision. Moreover, the results may be confounded by the effects of residency and fellowships on the graduates. Fourth, assessment of this goal relies on the use of historical controls (students in previous classes who were not exposed to the new curriculum) and thus cannot easily separate the effects of the new curriculum from trends in medicine as a whole.

Our discussions of the definition of "better physician" centered on qualities such as extensive and appropriate knowledge, humanism, compassion, career achievement, and the ability and desire to learn throughout life. Better physicians were thought to be more satisfied with the role of physician, especially as related to patient care, and more receptive to clinical research and academic medicine. We have used the results of AAMC exit questionnaires from a period of several years to examine trends in the attitudes of Johns Hopkins graduates toward clinical research, academic medicine, and patient care before and after implementation of the new curriculum. Methods of evaluating the humanistic qualities of physicians have been developed, but they are not feasible for us because they require either direct observation or surveys of colleagues and nursing staff.

As graduates of the new curriculum move into residency and professional practice, we intend to monitor their views of their education at Johns Hopkins. We hope to determine what they see as its strengths and weaknesses, and what they believe has been the impact of the new curriculum on their approaches to and attitudes toward learning and on their subsequent training and practice. We plan to assess other aspects of our graduates' practice patterns, as well, as they move beyond residency training. We are well aware of potential confounders. For example, if we find that more of our students are committed to general practice than in the past, should we attribute this to the increase in ambulatory care experiences at Johns Hopkins or to market forces?

Further answers to some of our questions will emerge from the AAMC exit questionnaire given to students in the last quarter of their fourth year. These questionnaires may also provide information about new issues that are raised as we continue to accumulate data from students who have completed the new curriculum.

We also intend to construct questionnaires for distribution to our graduates as they complete their first and third years of residency training. These questionnaires will focus on graduates' views of their preparation for graduate training. In addition, to the extent possible (e.g., with graduates who take a residency at Johns Hopkins or nearby), we would like to conduct focus groups to gain a deeper understanding of graduates' perceptions of their undergraduate medical education and their perspectives on our chosen indicators of success for the new curriculum.

The Johns Hopkins Precursors Study is a longitudinal, prospective study of

Johns Hopkins medical students that began in 1947. It has evaluated long-term outcomes for the classes of 1948 through 1964. In the course of the study, methods have been developed to assess physicians' specialty choice,[10] practice setting, career achievement,[11] job satisfaction,[12] work demand and control,[13] and a host of other work-related variables. These methods will be used for follow-up on more recent graduates to assess these and other outcomes and to compare the experiences of students under the new and old curricula.

The Johns Hopkins curriculum was revised to ensure that our students remain among the best medical school graduates in the nation. Our evaluation plan is modest, perhaps, as measured against those for other programs. However, we believe that it will help us to determine how well the goals of the new curriculum have been met.

Notes

1. J. Benbassat, "Practical issues in the evaluation of medical curricula," in *Essays on curriculum development and formulation in medicine,* ed. G. Page (report of the Second Cambridge Conference, University of British Columbia, 1989), 111–21.

2. G. T. Moore, A. S. Peters, S. D. Block, R. E. Feldman, M. J. D. Good, and B. Good, "Evaluation of 'Preparing Physicians for the Future: A Program in Medical Education,'" final report to the Robert Wood Johnson Foundation, December 1996.

3. J. Spooner, G. Bordage, J. DeMarchais, J. Guilbert, K. Hagenfeldt, B. Jolly, R. Laweuer, S. Obenshain, and P. Stillman, "Evaluation of curricula: The practice," in Page, *Essays on curriculum development,* 124.

4. Association of American Medical Colleges, *Physicians for the twenty-first century: The GPEP report,* report of the Panel on the General Professional Education of the Physician and College Preparation for Medicine (Washington, D.C.: Association of American Medical Colleges, 1984).

5. J. A. Sosa, P. P. Chang, and J. H. Shatzer, "Looking back: Involving multiple students' perspectives in basic science curricular revision" (poster presented in Innovations in Medical Education exhibit, Association of American Medical Colleges Annual Meeting, New Orleans, 1992).

6. P. P. Chang, J. A. Sosa, and J. H. Shatzer, "A Johns Hopkins model: Medical students validate the need for reform and ongoing evaluation," (poster presented in Innovations in Medical Education exhibit, Association of American Medical Colleges Annual Meeting, Boston, 1994).

7. Association of American Medical Colleges, *GPEP report;* and Association of American Medical Colleges, *ACME-TRI report: Educating medical students* (Washington, D.C.: Association of American Medical Colleges, 1992).

8. R. E. Marshall, "Measuring the medical school learning environment," *Journal of Medical Education* 53 (1978): 98–104; A. F. Rezler and V. Rezmovic, "The learning style

inventory," *Journal of Allied Health* 19 (1981): 26–34; and M. R. Brown and R. Mitchell, "The development of the cognitive behavior survey to assess medical student learning" (paper presented at the annual meeting of the American Educational Research Association, San Francisco, April 1992), respectively.

9. V. E. Velculescu, J. K. Hurt, S. E. Johnson, E. C. Hsiao, P. K. Wu, S. E. Martin, M. M. Dias, A. C. Wisler, L. A. Snyder, and H. P. Lehmann, "Student evaluation of the first year of the new curriculum" (report to the faculty of the Johns Hopkins University School of Medicine, Baltimore, 1993).

10. B. L. Rollman, L. A. Mead, N.-K. Wang, and M. J. Klag, "Medical specialty and the incidence of divorce: The Johns Hopkins Precursors Study," *New England Journal of Medicine* 336 (1997): 800–803.

11. F. L. Brancati, D. M. Levine, S. Margolis, L. A. Mead, D. Martin, and M. J. Klag, "Early predictors of career achievement in academic medicine," *JAMA* 267 (1992): 1372–76; P. L. Graves and C. B. Thomas, "Correlates of midlife career achievement among women physicians," *JAMA* 254 (1985): 781–87.

12. D. E. Ford, L. A. Mead, P. P. Chang, D. M. Levine, and M. J. Klag, "Depression predicts cardiovascular disease in men: The Precursors Study" (paper presented at the Sixty-seventh Scientific Session of the American Heart Association), *Circulation* 90 (1994): 1–614 (abstract).

13. J. B. Johnson, E. M. Hall, D. E. Ford, L. A. Mead, D. M. Levine, N.-K. Wang, and M. J. Klag, "The psychosocial work environment of physicians: The impact of demands and resources on job dissatisfaction and psychiatric distress in a longitudinal study of Johns Hopkins Medical school graduates," *Journal of Occupational and Environmental Medicine* 37 (1995): 1151–59.

10

Conclusions

Catherine D. De Angelis, M.D.

The purpose of this concluding chapter is to provide readers with some principles, or lessons, learned from the experience of planning, developing, implementing, and evaluating a new curriculum in one medical school and overseeing its operation. I am certain that readers could add other principles learned from their own personal experience in curriculum reform or from reading the various chapters in this book. The following are what I consider to be the major lessons I learned by working from the inside at all levels and throughout the process. Not surprisingly, some of the most important lessons came from unsuccessful ventures; this might be considered the first, or most basic, principle.

1. *Begin with centralized leadership and full support from the top.* The dean of the school of medicine must fully embrace the initiative and be visibly supportive. While it is impossible for any dean to spend the time necessary to institute curricular change, he or she must designate a representative at a high level in the dean's office who can assume ultimate responsibility for the curriculum. This person must be involved in all aspects of curricular change. The dean must make it clear at every opportunity that he or she considers the change of curriculum a very high priority. This means mentioning it as a priority in all appropriate forums and, as far as possible, rewarding the faculty who become heavily involved in the process. The dean's reports or updates to the trustees, to the university president, to the advisory boards and faculty councils, and to the public should include progress reports on the curriculum.

2. *Choose the right leaders.* Faculty leaders must be identified and given responsibility for each segment or program in the new curriculum. At Johns Hopkins one key leader was put in charge of each of the following at the very beginning: the first-year basic science curriculum, the second-year bridging sciences, the new Physician and Society course, the new Introduction to Clinical Medi-

cine course, the Clinical Epidemiology course, and each of the required clinical clerkships. (In most of the clerkships, directors already were in place.)

Many of the faculty leaders must be chosen for particular personality traits beyond those traditionally associated with leadership (such as management skills, organizational skills, clear thinking, sense of humor, thick skin, and high standing with peers). In choosing the person who would direct our Office of Medical Education Services, for example, I sought someone with an easygoing personality who would neither put off nor be put off by physicians and medical scientists. This was especially important because Johns Hopkins had never had an official "medical educator." (To gain a fuller understanding of this point, see chapter 2.) All faculty leaders must interact frequently with the individual who has overall responsibility for the curriculum, especially in the early stages. These interactions become less frequent and involve more people at a time as the curriculum becomes better established, but they must continue as long as the curriculum continues.

3. *Invite faculty at all levels to contribute to the process as early as possible.* It is the faculty who ultimately will determine the success of the venture. Once the leadership is established, all faculty members who will in any way be involved in the new curriculum must be encouraged to provide input, not only on content but on the process for change. All faculty members must have a key faculty leader with whom they can discuss the issues. Even those who are most skeptical about the change—indeed, especially those—must be heard and their ideas considered seriously. Some of our most successful teachers and strongest advocates began as skeptics. Moreover, many of their ideas proved to be invaluable.

4. *Don't wait until you have full agreement from everyone—it will never happen.* Academic centers are the professional homes of many—perhaps most—of the brightest and most creative people in their fields. Creativity requires an ability to challenge whatever is current. Therefore, it is to be expected that a certain fraction of the faculty will lack enthusiasm for any given idea, especially in the beginning. Some never will agree that the change was beneficial, no matter what the final outcome. The most you can hope for from such individuals is that they refrain from sabotaging the initiative. Fortunately, we had no saboteurs at Johns Hopkins; all of the naysayers became leaders or proponents, or remained essentially silent as progress was made. Remember that you'll win some and you'll lose some. However, it is essential to win many more than you lose.

5. *Don't wait until all details have been worked out, or you'll never implement the plan.* Once the objectives, goals, and implementation process are established, deadlines must be set for each segment, and those deadlines must be kept. No group is better at meeting deadlines than academicians. It may mean

working long hours as the deadline nears, but academicians know how to make it happen.

Keeping deadlines is especially important for the first curricular components that are implemented. At Johns Hopkins, the details of the first basic science module, Molecules and Cells, were barely planned when the faculty began teaching the course. The same was true of the first section of the Physician and Society course. While this was very stressful to the faculty members involved in the early courses, they rose to the challenge and developed some of the most successful components of the new curriculum.

Many people doubted that our time schedules could be met. That skepticism, especially from people outside the institution, provided an extra stimulus to our faculty. The faculty's efforts were rewarded not only by success in implementing their components on time but by the pleasure of reading our progress reports to the doubters.

6. *Fix it even if it ain't broke.* If you wait until the curriculum no longer works, you'll harm some students and your reputation. Furthermore, making changes because you have to is likely to be more costly and stressful. It is always better to prevent a problem than to solve it once it becomes a reality. This is not to say that all change is good, or that simply because you change something it will be better. On the contrary, careful planning is vital. It is necessary to decide what can be improved and to set objectives, develop methods to achieve them, and project costs.

Most curricula benefit from a careful review. I cannot understand why some faculty members who constantly seek to improve the status quo in their professional specialties are so resistant to change in the curriculum. My lack of understanding notwithstanding, it happens.

One positive aspect of curricular change is that it sends the message that teaching and education are important. As part of the process, time and additional resources are made available for the improvement of that aspect of the school's mission.

7. *Don't expect everything to work, especially on the first attempt.* As with most things in life, we learned about various new programs from experience. Some ideas and projects that seemed wonderful in planning did not work. Some of these were simply abandoned or were only partially retained. For example, we tried out a longitudinal (half-day weekly) continuity outpatient experience for a small group of third-year students. While the students and faculty rated it very highly, it required too much space and faculty time to be adopted for the entire class. In its place we instituted the required three-week Ambulatory Clerkship in Internal Medicine to augment the ambulatory experience in the other required clinical clerkships. The continuity experience is now an elective for a

limited number of students. While this may not be the best way to teach continuity care or ambulatory care, it is the best we can do for now. Incremental change is valuable.

Some programs required several trials before an agreed-upon program resulted. One example is the first year of the Physician and Society course. It took three years and three different approaches to produce the format that we adopted for repetition. As time goes on, still other approaches may be initiated.

Even the best ideas don't always work right the first time. Some of our most successful programs, courses, and individual classes emerged from repetition with only modest changes over time. An example is the first-year Introduction to Clinical Medicine course.

8. *Recognize and make use of students' expertise in curricular needs.* Just as each patient is an expert of sorts in his or her own illness, students have expertise in what they need. This is not to say that they make the final decisions regarding content or process, only that their input is invaluable in such decisions. Students involved in the planning of our new curriculum provided excellent information about content that they believed was missing or duplicated and about teaching methods and styles that they preferred. Our faculty valued their input and continue actively to seek student input in minor alterations of the new curriculum. I believe this is one reason for the excellent student attendance in almost all of our classes. Students know that the faculty values their contribution and that every class reflects this in some way. Of course, students do not all agree on the issues, but the faculty can use all of their opinions and ideas in deciding what and how to teach.

9. *Make faculty development an integral part of the curricular design.* Even the most facile and effective faculty require ongoing training, especially as new teaching methods are developed. Some training can take place in workshops or seminars specifically designed to update faculty on the latest teaching techniques, or on the tried-and-true ones. These formats are especially important for new techniques such as small-group teaching, in which students take the lead, and in the use of standardized patients. However, workshops and seminars alone are insufficient; regular feedback from medical educators, faculty peers, and students is essential and in some ways more effective. Workshops and seminars are time consuming and require attendance in settings where teacher-student roles are reversed. Many faculty are uncomfortable in such settings, especially at first, and resist being taught by medical educators who are neither physicians nor medical scientists. The "they're not like me" phenomenon sometimes makes it difficult for faculty to learn. Usually they are converted when it becomes clear that they are learning to be more effective teachers, but it can be difficult to draw them in. An ongoing relationship between faculty and medical educators and contin-

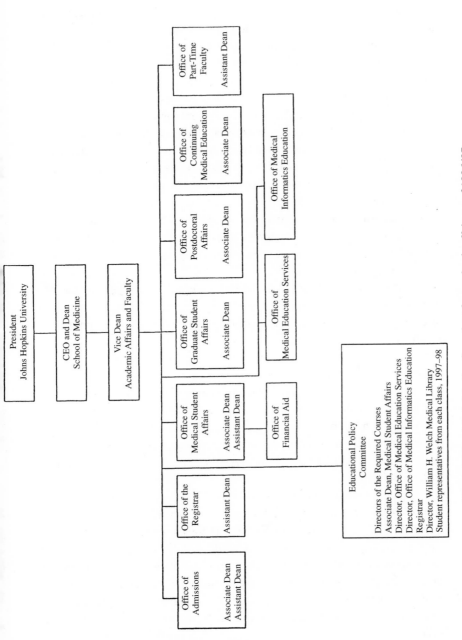

Figure 10.1 Administrative flow chart for academic affairs as of 1996/97

ued dialogue on teaching techniques through committees, program planning, and day-to-day activities are the best ways to engender faculty development.

10. *Remember that instituting a new curriculum requires new resources, primarily new funding and space.* It is useless to plan for a new curriculum or even a particular new program without ensuring that costs will be met and that sufficient space will be available. In our case, new monies were needed to support broad new programs like the Physician and Society course, to pay faculty for the additional work hours required by small-group sessions, and to hire new staff for the Office of Medical Education Services and the Office of Medical Informatics Education. New space was needed to house these offices and the new Clinical Education Center. In addition, the increased use of computers necessitated rewiring of laboratories and classrooms.

It is important to keep ahead of—or at least on—the curve of new developments in the field of curriculum design and implementation. Once you fall behind, it takes a much greater initiative and more money (or at least a larger sum at one time) to catch up.

11. *Before you start the process, determine how high-level barriers will be managed.* While considering whether to accept responsibility for the curricular change, I met with the dean to discuss the possibility of resistance from department directors and other leaders. I was already aware of the university president's support. The dean was strongly committed to providing administrative and financial support. He made his commitment to me clear when several basic science directors went directly to him because they believed that I wasn't providing sufficient funds to their departments. (I refer the reader to chapter 2 for a discussion of this issue.)

Throughout the process, the dean made it clear to everyone that the curriculum was a high priority in decisions regarding space, finances, and all other matters.

12. *Institutionalize the change process as a valued and extended endeavor rather than as a five-year project.* It is essential that an administrative process be established to provide conditioning support for the curriculum. Figure 10.1 shows the administrative flow chart for academic affairs at the medical school. The responsibility of the Educational Policy Committee to oversee all curricular change and all matters related to the curriculum (e.g., grading of students and evaluation of the overall curriculum and of individual programs) has been institutionalized. Any change would require an active and specific administrative decision from the dean.

Index